Trust Me,
I'm (Still) a Doctor

Also by Dr Phil Hammond

Medicine Balls

Trust Me, I'm (Still) a Doctor

Dr Phil Hammond

BLACK & WHITE PUBLISHING

First published 2008
by Black & White Publishing Ltd
29 Ocean Drive, Edinburgh EH6 6JL

1 3 5 7 9 10 8 6 4 2   08 09 10 11 12

ISBN 13:   978 1 84502 229 7

Typeset by RefineCatch Limited, Bungay, Suffolk
Printed and bound by MPG Books Ltd Bodmin, Cornwall

Thanks To

Jo, Will and Ellie
Miles Kington
Ian Hislop
Private Eye
Michael Mosley and the *Trust Me, I'm a Doctor* research team
The Observer
The Independent
Jan Poloniecki
Maria von Hildebrand
Ernest Codman
Heidi Beck
Black & White
and
all of my sources

CONTENTS

Introduction   ix

Blame the Tories   1
   Kenneth Clarke   5
   William Waldegrave   10
   Virginia Bottomley   21
   Stephen Dorrell   44

Blame Labour   57
   Frank Dobson   60
   Alan Milburn   110
   John Reid   180
   Patricia Hewitt   216
   Alan Johnson   255

Afterthoughts   293
   The Conscious Patient Guide   303
   Getting The Right Treatment Done Right   309
   Speak up Questions   314
   Harsh Truths   319
   Further Reading   320
   Cut out and Keep   321

INTRODUCTION
Unlucky Dip

'Knowledge is knowing that a tomato is a fruit.
Wisdom is knowing not to put one in a fruit salad.'

Miles Kington

It's 21 years since I qualified as a doctor, and I'm still amazed (and touched) that anyone should trust me. Most people would run a mile if someone ginger honed in on them with a cheesy come-hither grin (check the cover), but wearing a stethoscope somehow makes it alright. There are times when you have to trust a doctor, like when your blood pressure has fallen off the scale or there's a piece of bone sticking through your leg. But there are also times when it's worth asking the odd awkward question. Such as 'would you mind washing your hands first?', 'have you actually done this before?' or 'is this the best drug you've got, or merely the cheapest?'

Healthcare is a lucky dip. Our aim is to 'do the right thing right': spot the diagnosis quickly and give you the best available treatment with clean, steady hands and lashings of compassion. The reality is that medicine is complex and unpredictable, and there are lots of competing demands. Too many people get the wrong care – wrong diagnosis or treatment – or they get the right treatment wrongly given – delayed or bodged.

The NHS has traditionally blamed its shortcomings on lack of funding. Not having enough doctors, nurses, cleaners, drugs, training, sleep and machines that go ping adds up to a pretty dangerous mix. It's like climbing aboard a plane with a bit of wing missing, a hole in the fuselage and a pilot who's never flown before, who hasn't slept for 72 hours but is determined to 'have a go.' Miraculously, or rather because of the expertise and dedication of the staff, 90% of patients are 'satisfied' or 'very satisfied' with their NHS care. But it's not always a safe system to work or be ill in. 10% of patients and staff – often the unhappy ones – are damaged (physically and psychologically) by being in the NHS.

When I qualified in 1987, the 'training' mantra was 'see one, do one, teach one.' You'd see someone do a liver biopsy, either in the flesh or on *Casualty*, and off you'd pop with a large needle to have a go on some unwitting patient before teaching the next doctor how to do it. My first liver biopsy was a partial success with a very long needle – I got a bit of liver, a bit of spleen, a bit of kidney and a bit of bladder. More of a kebab, really. But the patient was effusively grateful: 'You've gotta learn somehow.'

There was so much dangerous dabbling, but no-one wanted to talk about it for fear of frightening patients. So I formed a double-act called *Struck Off and Die* with Tony Gardner and we tried it out about as far away from our workplace as we could find (the Edinburgh Fringe). It was more of a therapy session than a comedy, but it got us invited to a BBC Radio Light Entertainment Christmas party, where I followed the Beverley Sisters down the stairs and Ian Hislop into the toilet. I offered him a column for *Private Eye* and washed my hands afterwards.

I've been the *Eye*'s medical correspondent for 16½ years, and I'd like to think I've been a fierce advocate for a safer and fairer NHS. Unfortunately, no-one takes much notice of angry exposure in a satirical magazine written under a pseudonym (MD). As I've got older, and closer to being a patient, I've tried to move away from just exposing bad healthcare to understanding it. But not excusing it. We're now putting nearly £100 billion a year into the NHS and we deserve a good service for that money.

The bulk of this book is the distilled wisdom of over 400 *Private Eye* columns, originally published as *Doing the Rounds* and, more recently, *Medicine Balls*. The book is helpfully divided into 'Blame the Tories' and 'Blame Labour'. I've name-checked health secretaries to fill us with nostalgia (or nausea). Health secretary is seldom a good career move, and almost invariably ends in failure because you've stoked up expectations you can't hope to deliver in the time frame. So you panic and introduce wave upon wave of untested reforms that leave the staff giddy and bitter.

If the last 60 years have taught us anything about the NHS, it's that politicians shouldn't try to run it from Whitehall. Now Lord Darzi – Labour Health Minister and everyone's favourite robot-assisted surgeon – has decided to put doctors back in charge, encouraging us (not me, personally) to go for every top management job.

So can doctors be trusted, once again, to run the NHS? Certainly more so than politicians. Especially if they work in teams with other professionals, accepting criticism and knowing the limits of their competence. In the last 16½ years, I've exposed enough medical scandals to make your head explode. These aren't exclusively the fault of doctors, but just hammer home the point that doctors are human. We may be very bright and reasonably ethical, but if you put us in an unsafe, underfunded and unaccountable NHS and throw in a touch of arrogance and self-interest, it can pretty soon turn pear-shaped.

Doctors are their own harshest critics and many of the stories I've written about have come from whistleblowing medics. I've also met those on the receiving end of medical accidents, which has stoked up my anger but also provided inspiration. Most don't want to blame and sue, but to understand what happened and prevent it happening to someone else.

The biggest scandal I've uncovered is the Bristol heart disaster, but the NHS at that time was full of 'Bristols' – staff with inadequate resources and expertise getting bad results but struggling on regardless because there was no mechanism to help or stop them.

I hope the NHS is safer because of what happened in Bristol, but as only heart surgeons publish their results it's very hard to tell. A lot of our money now seems to go to shareholders, rather than safety. As the late Paul Foot put it: 'there has been an enormous transfer of power in Britain from public, elected authorities to private, unelected corporations.' And they don't invite scrutiny.

After the Bristol inquiry in 2001, Labour had a real opportunity to put quality and safety at the heart of the health service, but Tony Blair soon tired of that and decided instead to feed the NHS to the market. Unfair competition, commercial secrecy, duplication of services, distrust of management, job insecurity, intimidation, bullying and an obsession with profitability are not the ingredients of safe healthcare. Everyone who works in the Department of Health and the NHS should (re)read the Bristol inquiry report, or at least the summary, and get back on track.

This is my contribution to the debate, charting my journey from lean, angry stand-up junior doctor to fat, angry sit-down GP. One of the delights (and embarrassments) of performing comedy is that you get immediate feedback, good or bad. But in medicine, outcomes are much harder to measure, and often we don't bother, so you could be a mass-murdering GP and still have a heaving (but slowly diminishing) waiting room.

The Tories and Labour are now falling over themselves to publish outcomes. Hopefully not just crude death statistics and meaningless league tables, but more subtle stuff that involves talking to patients and finding out if they can still hop and skip a year after their hip replacement or heart surgery. 'Patient-reported outcomes' are becoming all the rage and require feedback from those on the receiving end, which can only be a good thing.

In an ideal world, we'd assemble all these outcomes, adjust

them for risk to make sure those treating sicker patients are fairly represented, and then compare one team's figures with the average of all the other teams' figures in the UK, for each procedure. If a unit fell below an agreed safety standard (e.g. double the average mortality or complication rate elsewhere), this would prompt a swift investigation (in a supportive, grown-up way) to find out why (and to protect patients).

Unfortunately, the Government and medical establishment aren't rushing to set standards, perhaps because they're worried they might be sued by those who don't reach them. So publication is going ahead and it's left to patients to decide their own standards. Do you want to go to hospital X which is on your doorstep with cheap coffee and easy parking and a mortality rate for your operation of 16%? Or do you want to travel 50 miles to hospital Y where you don't know anyone and you couldn't afford to park even if you could find a space, but the mortality rate is 4%? It's called patient choice.

One of Labour's key reforms, 'Shifting the Balance of Power', is known in the Department of Health as 'Shifting the Blame onto Patients'. Now that patients have 'choice', they have to accept responsibility when things go wrong. I think this is cruel and not terribly wise, but that's politics for you. It's never been a tougher time to be a patient. So I've concluded this book with a 'Conscious Patient Guide' for those outside the anaesthetic who want to ask the odd awkward question if only they could think of one.

There's also a cut-out-and-keep membership card for the Royal College of Patients, for you to display prominently on your bedside locker or handbag. It's a virtual organisation that I've founded to take on the might of the medical establishment. Everyone is a vice president, whether you want to be one or not. There is no president but I'm thinking of asking Helen Mirren to be the Royal Patron. No matter how much money we put into the NHS, it will only get safer and better if patients find their voice: 'As Vice President of the Royal College of Patients,

I was wondering how likely it is that you're going to kill me?' It might just make all the difference. Good luck, and let me know how it goes.

Dr Phil

August 2008

drphil@bbc.co.uk

PS: Some of these stories featured in previous editions of *Trust Me, I'm a Doctor* (1999, 2001 – both now out of print) and in the BBC TV series of the same name. But one thing I've learned as a journalist, especially in a satirical magazine, is that you have to keep banging on with the same message for decades before anyone takes any notice. And it's not very good for your blood pressure.

The dates coincide with when a column was written, rather than the date of publication in *Private Eye*, and the articles may differ slightly from the edited versions that went to press. Anything that appears under the heading 'Notes' is where I've tried to shoehorn in some context, hindsight and self-justification.

Dr Phil's Notes

My first reflection on reading this book is that it revolves a lot around doctors, particularly surgeons, and especially those in Bristol. 90% of NHS activity has nothing to do with hospitals and most of it is administered by people who don't have a medical degree. Indeed, most healthcare goes on at home, where people use common sense to realise that illness often gets better through love and evolution, not antibiotics. However, hospitals do suck up most NHS funding, and weeding out ineffective, substandard and dangerous care should free up more money to stop us going into hospital in the first place. That's the theory . . .

BLAME THE TORIES
1988–1997

BLAME THE TORIES

I entered medical school in 1981, two years into Thatcher's first term and a year after the Black Report which nailed home the point that poor people get sick, and that the best way to improve health is to conquer poverty. Thatcher promptly buried it.

Norman Fowler was in charge of the Department of Health and Social Security for all my student years (1981–87), and somehow managed to prevent Thatcher from privatising the NHS. In 1986, he launched a memorable 'AIDS: Don't Die Of Ignorance' campaign (or 'ADIS: Don't Die Of Dyslexia', as the posters were changed to). Despite a speech impediment, Fowler gamely tried to lecture us on the importance of proper condom usage, a message lost on Cecil Parkinson, and kicked off the first in a long line of over-hyped health scares by stressing the point that 'everyone is at risk' from HIV infection. Leaflets were promptly dispatched to 23 million households, half of which contained either an elderly couple or an old person living alone. As one elderly, hypothermic Dorset woman commented in the *Guardian* (January 15, 1987): 'Do you think this caring government would swap my AIDS leaflet (as new) for a bucket of coal?' Better still, pile them high and burn them to keep warm.

The most profound change of the Fowler era completely passed me by as a student. Thatcher invited Sainsbury's chief Roy Griffiths to reform the NHS and he announced, in 1983, that we needed general managers at every level of the service. Anyone who couldn't get a job in a supermarket promptly jumped ship to the NHS. The health service clearly needs excellent management, but the Tory appointees were a mixed bag intent on burying bad news and bad debt, and silencing dissenters. In such a climate, quality and safety could never flourish.

KENNETH CLARKE
July 1988–November 1990

Fat Ken became health secretary on the back of a funding crisis, but fought off Tory plans to scrap the NHS and replace it with an insurance-based system. Instead, he utilised his new army of managers to reform the service along business lines, arguing that an internal market would somehow improve productivity and reduce costs. The NHS was divided into 'purchasers' and 'providers', and money was supposed to follow the patient anywhere he or she wished to travel. Alas, block contracts soon stopped any freedom of movement. The purchasers ran out of money every winter and the providers stopped treating patients, unless they happened to be those of GP fundholders, who seemed to have more money than everyone else.

Clarke claims to have come up with the idea of fundholding on the back of an envelope whilst in the bath, relaxing in a gentleman's way (or something like that). He wound up some GPs by telling them: 'Every time I mention the word reform, you reach for your wallet,' and annoyed them further by suggesting what they should do with their time. But entrepreneurial GPs grasped the nettle, improved the care of their patients and pocketed the profits.

Clarke was an unrepentant beer-and-cigarillos jazz buff. His dedication to the nation's health was further questioned when he became deputy chairman of British American Tobacco and voted against the smoking ban. Fellow MP Alan Clark called him 'a puffball' and 'a pudgy life-insurance risk', but Clarke survived Clark. Managers loved him for leaving them alone to get on with commercialising healthcare. Lots of beans were counted and boxes ticked, but the NHS still seemed pretty dangerous to me.

THE INDEPENDENT
Fringe Medics Show Death Wish

10 August 1990   By Miles Kington

My Edinburgh withdrawal symptoms are quite severe this year. Having been involved in most of the last 15 fringes, I badly need that dose of adrenaline, camaraderie, excitement, dirty socks and staying up far too late for fear of missing something. Last year I was with *Instant Sunshine* at the Pleasance for two weeks. This year, nowhere.

What makes it worse is that for the last three months I have been getting posters and leaflets for Edinburgh Fringe shows through my letterbox. As, however, I am a hard-eyed monster of egoism, and jealous of anyone actually going there, I have remained totally unaffected by these Fringe hopefuls.

With one exception. Phil Hammond, a junior doctor from Bristol, is going up with a fellow doctor, Tony Gardner, to do two things of such extraordinary difficulty that even to attempt them smacks of a death wish. He clearly needs all the help he can get.

The first is to rescue the good name of medical humour. Every year, medical student groups go to Edinburgh with material that might provoke hoots of laughter at the hospital Christmas show, but is groaned off the stage in the real world. Shows with names such as *Medicine Balls*, *The Enema Within* and *Just a Little Prick*.

Well, medics have to deal with the crude side of life, so their escape from it is equally crude. When you are the one made responsible for pain and misery, it is wonderful to be irresponsible for a while. Those doctors who rise above it into

6

other levels of humour (J Miller, G Garden and R Buckman) have usually escaped from medicine as well.

The extraordinary thing in medical humour is that one target is never aimed at. The doctors themselves. The whole medical set-up. The whole crazy, overworked, underfunded, killingly tired, hierarchical, nepotistic health service is never got at. You can make jokes about bowels and rubber tubing, but never about drunken consultants or doctors getting a commission from cremation forms. Hammond and Gardner reckon they are the first doctors in the revue field to rise above lavatorial level and have a go at the way medicine is run in this country. Two, as I say, hard targets.

I know just how hard it is because when I first teamed up with *Instant Sunshine* twenty years ago, the other three were still junior doctors and absolutely terrified that playing with such a group would ruin their careers; afraid senior doctors would get the impression that they were not serious chaps. I was in charge of writing concert and programme notes, when needed. For 10 years they would not let me mention their medical connections, which, as they were (and are) full-time doctors left not a lot to talk about.

It was a ludicrous situation. It was ludicrous that when they went for job interviews, they were scared stiff that one of the panel might have seen them playing. It was ludicrous that junior doctors who were not even guilty of criticising the regime (they thought much of the system asinine, but went along with it in the same way as chaps at boarding school do) felt they had to behave as if they were.

'How do your doctors make time for *Instant Sunshine*?' people ask me.

'They let their patients die,' I tell them.

This is not true. It is junior doctors working for 80 hours non-stop who have to let their patients die. But Hammond is the first medic to get up on stage and get a laugh by saying so. There is a chance he might be putting his job on the line. In many medical contracts, there is an extraordinary clause forbidding doctors to talk to the Press. There is, as far as I know, no medical contract which says the doctor may not go to Edinburgh and there make fun of his employers on the stage, but there doesn't really need to be. Not in the medical profession.

I haven't met Hammond or seen the act, but I like the sound of someone who, because junior doctors get less than £2 an hour overtime, hands out badges to the audience that read 'I earn more than my doctor.' I like someone who says: 'The reason we draw the curtains when a patient dies is so the doctor can raid the fruit bowl without anyone seeing.' I'd like to think he sells out at Venue 6, Celtic Lodge, Brodie's Close, Lawnmarket, 12–25 August inclusive, from midnight to 1.15am. Good luck, lads.

Struck Off and Die
Programme Notes

August 1990

Struck Off and Die are two tired and surly junior doctors, Tony Gardner and Phil Hammond, who got together to publicise our working conditions and wage a war of ridicule on the medical establishment. We encourage criticism (and chocolates) and are especially keen to hear from anyone who has felt the rough end of the NHS pineapple (confidentiality assured, all letters answered, photo appreciated). Concessions for this show are available for NHS staff and the relatives of anyone we've killed. Sorry.

Some Facts
• Junior doctors work on average 90 hours per week (Dowie 1989).

- Every third week, most work a continuous 81-hour shift for which a house officer earns less than £2 an hour before tax.
- The CEPOD Report (1987) highlighted 140 preventable surgical deaths at the hands of overtired, unsupervised juniors. Ennis and Vincent (1990) found that human error and lack of supervision were at the heart of 64 obstetric disasters.
- Drug addiction rates amongst doctors are 30 times the national average and they are three times as likely to die of cirrhosis and four times as likely to commit suicide. No figures are available for church attendance.
- Less than 1% of consultant surgeons are women, and only 6% of physicians. It doesn't help if you're black, either.

Thought For The Day: Is killing patients when you're tired – and then killing yourself – the only way to learn?

WILLIAM WALDEGRAVE
November 1990–April 1992

William Waldegrave took over when John Major came to power, and told a reporter he'd 'rather be back in the Foreign Office'. Waldegrave never seemed comfortable as health secretary, nor with a commercialised NHS. As he put it: 'The NHS market isn't a market in the real sense . . . it's competition in the sense that there will be comparative information available.' Alas, the comparative information was largely about cost and productivity, and not anything that told patients about the quality and safety of their care.

Patients could still use the press to raise questions about the NHS, but Waldegrave wasn't too keen on that either. On March 23, 1992, in the run-up to the election, he sent a letter to the editors of regional newspapers: 'I write to urge immense caution in the use of individual case histories where the NHS is alleged to have failed a patient. Very many of the individual cases alleged have, on investigation, turned out either to be completely false or heavily distorted.' He then disappeared into the ether.

I stood against him in that election for the Struck Off and Die Junior Doctors' Alliance (SODJA), but I only met him at the count when he vaguely suggested we could meet up for a chat about my concerns (possibly knowing that he wouldn't be health secretary any more). The Bristol heart scandal was going on in his constituency, under his nose, but he was relieved to get out of the Department of Health relatively unscathed.

PRIVATE EYE

17 January 1992

It's an unhappy new year all round for those working in health secretary William Waldegrave's beleaguered NHS. . . .

In Bloomsbury, junior doctor Chris Johnstone has won the right to sue his health authority for subjecting him to a particularly onerous obstetrics job, and little progress has been made on cutting doctors' hours. Johnstone took his decision after falling asleep at the wheel. He used a portable brain wave monitor to measure his cerebral activity during a 48-hour shift, and found that he was registering sleep waves while sewing up women after labour. Despite his high court victory, the job remained the same and the doctor who followed him spent time in intensive care after a paracetamol overdose.

The Government is trying to reduce junior doctors' hours in the most intensive jobs to just 83 per week without employing any more doctors. Forcing the same number of doctors to do the same amount of work in less time will be even more dangerous than the present system. The deal itself can only be saved if consultants agree to make up the shortfall in manpower. Meanwhile, a year after the deal was announced, surgical house officers in Newcastle are working 150 hours a week to cover for colleagues on holiday.

14 February 1992

In health secretary William Waldegrave's home city, managers at the United Bristol Healthcare Trust have come up with a novel way to cut waiting lists. Since all operations, however trivial, are counted together, list reductions have been achieved by concentrating on tiny plastic procedures. Lorry loads of 'bat ears', some of whom had been waiting for more than 10 years, were pinned back en masse at the expense of more substantial operations that took longer – a triumph of numbers over need.

With Mr Major's two-years-or-less waiting list promise looming, NHS managers are desperate to farm operations out to local private hospitals. Some private patients currently reach theatre without being examined and, with just one doctor resident in most private hospitals, the level of post-operative supervision is, er, not all it might be. And if shit happens, there isn't a cardiac arrest team close at hand. As many of the NHS patients are likely to be elderly, and a lot sicker than your average private patient, one can only hope that no-one suffers in this efficiency drive.

The current record for NHS understaffing is held by Manor Park Hospital, also in Bristol, where a single on-call junior doctor has to look after 360 geriatric in-patients, some of whom are very ill, sprawled over eighteen wards. Plymouth comes a close second, where one doctor is expected to minister to sick geriatric patients in three busy hospitals at once. The job includes the traditional 81-hour continuous shift, known locally as 'suicide weekend'.

Many NHS staff contracts have now been doctored to include an intimidating 'loyalty clause' effectively forbidding freedom of speech. Staff who do speak out are being shown the door. A leaked managerial document from Trent aimed to end the 'paranoia and posturing of rival professional groups' by sacking 'renegades and subversives.' Ouch.

In Cheltenham, the on-call room for the anaesthetist covering the intensive care unit has been helpfully moved to the far end of the hospital, well outside the two-minute emergency-sprinting distance. And down in the Special Care Baby Unit, senior house officers with no paediatric experience have no emergency back-up either, apart from a consultant-at-home. One junior was told he'd need to 'fly by the seat of his pants' if he got the job.

28 February 1992

The Royal Gwent in Newport, like many other district general hospitals, employs inexperienced junior doctors to cover the Special Care Baby Unit and labour wards with only a consultant-at-home for back-up. The unit turns-over 4,500 babies a year, all of whom require oxygen to the brain well before the 30 minutes it takes a paediatrician to arrive in an emergency. One doctor was left alone to ventilate a 28-week-old baby on a new machine with an instruction manual in German. Meanwhile, in Chepstow, junior plastic surgeons are clocking up 100 hours a week, a mere ten years after attempts to abolish such rotas.

13 March 1992

The King's Fund's observation that London's health system is 'near collapse' is a tad at odds with William Waldegrave's rosy prediction. Many inner-London hospitals charge at least 30% extra for routine treatments to subsidise their large quota of emergency and super-specialist work. Not surprisingly, they aren't faring too well in the Tories' internal market and are desperate to save money.

Managers at the Royal London Hospital Trust have cut community psychiatric nursing and other essential services by £250,000 to bail out emergency work. At King's Hospital, some patients have been stuck in the corridor for 36 hours and a few have died-in-waiting. Understaffing of intensive care beds has long caused avoidable deaths as very sick patients are nursed on general wards without adequate observation.

Delayed admissions and inadequate in-patient care of cancer patients at London's St Bartholomew's Hospital has led to the resignation of Mr Jerry Gilmore, a senior cancer surgeon. And the low media profile of psychiatric patients has allowed Victorian asylums to be run down en masse. Hackney Hospital recently won an award for 'worst psychiatric hospital in Britain' and consultant Dr Niall Moore has volunteered to bulldoze it down. Unfortunately, lack of community care means the alternative for many psychiatric patients is to be knocked down on a zebra crossing.

Community care continues to suffer from its 'insensitivity to the market' (although it won't be long before managers are pricing empathy). At Bexley Hospital in Kent, the intended closure of Elmdene Alcoholic Unit would deprive the area of a vital centre for detoxification, education and support. There simply isn't any profit in it.

27 March 1992

When a BBC Radio Bristol reporter asked William Waldegrave how he felt about taking over as health secretary, his reply was telling: 'I'd rather be back in the Foreign Office.' Today, a glance at the hospitals in his Bristol West constituency will do little to change his mind.

Recent reports of Bristol Children's Hospital demanding a cash pledge from Worcester Royal Infirmary before allowing a critically injured child through its doors may have caused ructions in the national press, but for those working in Bristol, it hardly raised an eyebrow. The Bristol Royal Infirmary (BRI) has a long-standing 'bed crisis' in intensive care because managers have persistently refused to provide the specialist staff needed to service more than five beds.

In the last four months, 94 patients have been refused an intensive care bed and 40% have subsequently died. Patients who have the misfortune to miss out are nursed on general wards, often by agency nurses with no specialist training. But despite the lack of beds, the rush to beat the April waiting-list deadline has meant that vascular surgeons are continuing to do major cases, such as aneurysm repairs, without post-operative intensive care.

On the weekend of February 22 and 23, the situation became farcical. The intensive care unit was again full. Two patients, surrounded by their distraught relatives, were artificially ventilated in the recovery room of an emergency operating theatre, blocking its use. Several other would-be intensive care patients were nursed on general wards and at least two requiring ventilation didn't get it. One patient who was bleeding from an ulcer would 'in an ideal world have had surgery', according to her doctor. She was denied it because she would have required intensive care post-op. Every surgeon has now received a memo asking them not to operate on any patient who may need intensive care afterwards.

THE OBSERVER
Junior, Behave Yourself

28 June 1992

Should you feel sorry for junior doctors? You don't see many of us with rickets. Most come from cosy professional backgrounds and go on to earn healthy sums of money in secure jobs with satisfaction and respect. And a few are so insufferably arrogant, it's hard for the rest to engender mass sympathy.

True, I could fill this column with horror stories of patients dying at the hands of tired, abused and unsupervised doctors, or of promising careers ending prematurely in alcoholism or suicide, but how much of that is self-inflicted? It's easy to blame 'the system' for a doctor's lot, but the system is largely composed of other doctors and we never were very good at accepting the buck. 'Bury the notes and burn the X-rays' is the stock solution to another tired cockup.

After five years fighting a futile hours-reduction battle that started when I was in nappies, one question still perplexes me. How can a profession that purports to care for patients have so little regard for its own? The vast majority of consultants are not knowingly abusive towards their junior staff. True, there is a countrywide smattering of childishly malevolent surgeons who could do with an empathy infusion, but many more well-meaning specialists still suffer from a huge reality gap.

Most of us communicate badly with patients because we've never been poor, sick, black or even female. But even when we've experienced the iniquities of medical training first hand, it's all too easy to progress into consultant-hood with the misguided air of 'it didn't do me any harm.' Besides, if you've sacrificed your marriage and your liver to make it to the top, you don't want the bastards beneath you to find an easier route.

And after a few whiskies in the clubby locker-room atmosphere of an all-male common room, you tend to view your formative years through blood-tinted spectacles: 'We used to work for weeks on end ... never saw daylight ... and I enjoyed every minute of it.' Blah, blah, blah. Long hours weren't quite so onerous when the only therapeutic options were Horlicks or extra potatoes.

Technology, turnover and patient expectation have risen so sharply that few consultants have any idea what life's like on the bottom rung today. And with the administration, intimidation and uncertainty of the reforms, none of them has the stamina to find out.

Perhaps junior doctors deserve the mess they're in. Too many of us would rather sacrifice our own and our patients' well-being than stand up for ourselves. The combination of apathy, fear and fatigue has never allowed us to present a united front. 'Give us what we want or a handful of us will get in a strop' is unlikely to cut much ice with the Tories.

It would be nice to have a well-organised union behind us but we're stuck with the BMA. The traditional public school bias of medicine has bred a self-perpetuating profession of sheltered, spoon-fed sycophants with as much independent thought as a decerebrate baboon.

Though medical schools now accept students from a broader base, the mould remains to be broken: you don't see many black or female faces in a Royal College of Surgeons' group photo. Assured of success, the 'white, male and hearty' brigade have no need to rock the boat. Anyone else dare not. 'You're only as good as your last reference' is the familiar cry of the downtrodden doctor. Moving from job to job every six months, our futures depend on the vagaries of successive consultants. Tough luck if you end up with Sir Lancelot Spratt.

The only possible way out of this mess is for the profession to accept its share of the blame. The problem isn't simply one of hours. There's a long-standing cycle of self-inflicted abuse that has become so ingrained into junior doctor culture that even patients cease to be shocked by it.

The cycle will be impossible to break without a simultaneous overhaul of our training. The restrictive and secretive practices of the Royal Colleges must be replaced with openly restructured and team-based training, so that a whimsical prejudice doesn't mean the end of a promising career. Consultant selection must have more to do with clinical competence and less to do with trouser legs.

Training should be centred on one area, so doctors can establish a home base and a low-alcohol social life, and learn to fight their ground with consultants and managers alike. And working conditions should be well publicised so juniors can shop around for humane jobs while unpleasant ones remain unfilled.

None of this is likely to happen overnight. The Government, too, has become so blinkered that many long-term improvements are being sacrificed on the ill-advised altar of waiting lists *über alles*. But only tradition bars doctors from being supportive of each other. And if we swallowed our egos, we'd get a lot more sympathy.

Dr Phil's Notes

I've never totally recovered from my angry junior doctor phase, but it peaked after about five years. During that time, I was photographed dropping a baby for the *Sunday Times Magazine*, I threatened to take junior doctors out on strike in Jersey, I picketed the Tory conference in Blackpool and I stood for parliament against the health secretary William Waldegrave.

I took Waldegrave to the wire in Bristol West, creaming off 87 votes to his 22,169. In retrospect, hiring an ice-cream van as a campaign bus and driving around the streets of Clifton shouting 'What do we want? Willie Out! When do we want it? Now!' was never going to get me elected. The futility of using comedy to change anything was driven home by Harvey Thomas, Margaret Thatcher's campaign manager, who told me: 'You're a medical kook. If you want to be taken seriously, you have to be serious.' Doesn't seem to be working for Gordon Brown, though. You need optimism and a smile that doesn't frighten children too.

Comedy exists purely to make people laugh. You can't save the NHS with it, because you can never be sure why people are laughing. When I stood on stage at Edinburgh and said 'my local heart surgery unit is known as the Killing Fields and the Departure Lounge,' people roared with laughter. Doctors seemed to think it was particularly funny, and even if a few of them thought 'there's something not quite right going on there,' they weren't going to do anything about it. Their emotional response was to laugh, and having done that, they could move on to the next scary story.

Displacing your emotions into satire and black humour happens a lot in medicine. Every hospital has a surgeon known affectionately as 'Butcher' or 'Hacker' or even 'The Terminator'. Bristol boasted a heart surgeon called 'Killer' long before the heart scandal. But very few people blow the whistle or act to protect patients, although they might try to ensure their friends and family are diverted elsewhere. Even though Tony and I were outraged by our dangerous working conditions, I suspect *Struck Off and Die* reinforced as many attitudes as we changed. You can judge for yourself in a chapter tucked away near the end of *Medicine Balls*.

My medical hero is an American surgeon called Ernest Codman, who tried to change the world with passion and sincerity: 'I am called eccentric for saying in public that hospitals, if they wish to be sure of improvement, must find out what their results are, must analyse their results to find their strong and weak points, must compare their results with those of other hospitals, must care for what cases they can care for well, and avoid attempting to care for cases which they are not qualified to care for well. They must welcome publicity not only for their successes, but for their errors. Such opinions will not be eccentric a few years hence.' And that was in 1910.

Codman was, and still is, spot on. To have any idea if anything works in medicine, you have to measure outcomes and that means doing post-mortems on the dead to find out why they died, and talking to the living to find out if you've made any difference to their lives. The best part of *Struck Off and Die* was in the bar afterwards where other doctors would tell shocking stories we could nick, but patients too would share their experiences. Many loved the NHS, but some had a dreadful time. Slowly the penny dropped, and I shifted from defending doctors to protecting patients.

The pious *Observer* piece was deservedly rude about the medical establishment. I couldn't understand how a profession that was so intelligent and influential couldn't get its act together over junior doctors' hours. They did eventually come down (some say by too much), and the junior doctors who campaigned the hardest are now beleaguered consultants working harder than ever to cover their junior staff, who knock off as soon as their shift is over. Back in 1992, the working conditions of the NHS could be hell for all doctors, junior and senior alike. And when you're so wound up in your own hardship, it can be easy to lose sight of patients.

VIRGINIA BOTTOMLEY
1992–1995

Gorgeous, pouting Virginia Hilda Brunette Maxwell Bottomley was known to her colleagues as Nanny, because of her fondness for health promotion. She saw her role as a custodian rather than a politician, to bed-in the Tory reforms: 'In politics you sometimes want a window-breaker and sometimes a glazier. Ken Clarke was definitely a window-breaker and I'm much more a glazier.'

She made the old farts in the British Medical Association swoon, and they gave her a standing ovation for instigating a deal to reduce junior doctors' hours (though not quickly enough for me). She also increased medical school numbers just before she left office. She didn't seem that keen on markets either, and in her valedictory speech, she extolled the virtues of planning and collaboration.

I've met her twice, once at the Hospital Doctor of the Year Awards in 1992, when she fretted that the winner might come from a London hospital that was earmarked for closure in the Tomlinson review. And once at a BUPA 60th Anniversary Celebration, when she didn't laugh at any of my jokes but I flogged her a couple of copies of *Medicine Balls* (replete with the unfortunate anagram of her name – I'm an evil Tory bigot).

Bottomley struck me as terribly earnest and well-meaning, but a bit too close to doctors, perhaps because she has them in her family. Like Waldegrave before her, she didn't seem to notice the Bristol heart scandal, even though parents wrote to her for advice in 1992. The Government could pour public money into a failing, dangerous service without taking any responsibility for the outcome.

The Bristol Heart Disaster
1992

Dr Phil's Notes

The Bristol heart disaster was one of the first stories I broke in *Private Eye* and it became the subject of the largest public inquiry in UK history, just seven years later. It finally forced the NHS to at least think about quality and safety, although this momentum was lost when they disappeared up the arse of Labour's competitive and secretive NHS market. At the time of writing, I didn't distinguish Bristol from any other example of dangerous care within the NHS. Thousands of people died (and still die) unnecessarily each year, and Bristol was only different in that it was babies rather than, say, old people.

Bristol hospitals were unfairly over-represented when I started writing for *Private Eye*, because I was living there and had lots of good sources. Only one has ever been brave enough to go public, the anaesthetist Stephen Bolsin, who paid for his concerns with his career and is now practising, very successfully, in Australia. Bolsin told the Bristol inquiry that he gave me information about the heart surgery unit as a concerned professional, and had no idea I wrote for *Private Eye*. So what follows is all my fault.

What vexed me in 1992 was not just that those in authority knew what was happening in Bristol and didn't act, but that the hospital management had the gall to pursue an award from the Department of Health while protecting a dangerous child heart surgery unit.

PRIVATE EYE

8 May 1992

Before the Department of Health bestows its mark of excellence on the United Bristol Healthcare Trust, it may wish to ponder the perilous state of its paediatric cardiac surgery. In 1988, the mortality was so high that the unit was dubbed 'The Killing Fields'. Despite a long crisis of morale among intensive care staff, the surgeons persistently refuse to publish their mortality rates in a manner comparable to other units. And although Dr Roylance (the chief executive) and the Department of Health are well aware of the problems, they won't recognise them officially.

Recently, the unit failed to provide a paediatric cardiac surgery nurse for post-operative care because it was assumed the baby would not survive the operation. And although Liverpool surgeons have successfully operated on 160 babies with Fallot's tetralogy, a congenital heart abnormality, the Bristol mortality rate is between 20% and 30%. Hardly the stuff of commendations.

3 July 1992

Health secretary Mrs Bottomley claims that whistleblowing 'through the correct channels' will get results. Staff at the United Bristol Healthcare Trust (UBHT) have been whistling about the dismal mortality statistics in the paediatric cardiac surgery unit since 1988. And while UBHT's chief executive John Roylance, the Royal College of Surgeons and the NHS Management Executive are well aware of the problem, they seem more concerned with silencing the blowers.

In America, the mortality rate for arterial switch, an operation to connect congenitally transposed arteries from the heart is now 0%. Nearer to home in Birmingham it is 3%. In Bristol, despite the fact that the operation has been performed since 1988, it is 30%. Sadly, consultant cardiologists at the Bristol Children's Hospital continue to refer patients to their surgeons to support the local unit. As a recently retired and very eminent cardiac surgeon in Southampton says: 'Everyone knows about Bristol.'

9 October 1992

The sorry state of paediatric cardiac surgery at the United Bristol Healthcare Trust has been confirmed by an internal audit of the last two years' operations. The results of procedures to correct two congenital abnormalities (Tetralogy of Fallot and transposition of the arteries) were especially poor. James Wisheart, chairman of the hospital management committee and medical adviser to the Trust board, is required to maintain standards of medical practice at UBHT. Curiously he has not felt it necessary to inform the Trust board or the Trust's purchasers of these findings. Could it be because he is also associate director of cardiac surgery?

20 November 1992

At the Bristol Royal Infirmary, part of the United Bristol Healthcare Trust (UBHT), ward closures and patient transfers have made the surviving wards look full, thus giving the impression that business is booming. Such imaginative management has resulted in UBHT being awarded a charter mark, despite its precarious paediatric cardiac surgery unit. All-day celebrations were generously sponsored by the trustees and a commemorative lapel badge is being commissioned for staff to wear with pride. Curiously, UBHT just happens to be in the middle of former health secretary William Waldegrave's constituency.

Letter Printed in *Private Eye*

18 December 1992

Sir,

I see that you are having another swipe at Bristol Royal Infirmary's 'precarious' paediatric cardiac surgery unit. Exactly what your objections to this unit are escape me, but I feel moved to write in its defence. Our son, born with Down Syndrome and congenital heart disease, was operated on at BRI last November to repair his hole in the heart. Every member of the staff showed an unswerving dedication to all aspects of Joseph's operation, including helping us, his family, through the most traumatic experience we have ever known.

I have heard it suggested that some hospitals are not prepared to carry out such an operation if the child concerned has Down Syndrome, as the risk of failure is too high. (This may be only unfounded rumour, so is likely to appear as fact in your next issue, no doubt.) Since the majority of children with Down Syndrome have such a heart defect with associated operative risk, those hospitals that are prepared to carry out the operation may well appear way down the list in a league table of success v. failure. However, what is the true story behind the bald statistics? Leave the BRI, or at least the cardiac unit, alone. Without it and all its staff, our son would be ill and dying. He is fit and healthy only because of them.

Yours faithfully,
Jeremy Doyle
Kingswear, Dartmouth

Dr Phil's Notes

Although the Bristol unit enjoyed some success, the public inquiry concluded that a third of the children who underwent open-heart surgery between 1984 and 1995 received 'less than adequate care' and in one four-year period alone (1991 to 1995) 'between 30 and 35 more children under one year died after open-heart surgery in the Bristol Unit than might be expected had the Unit been typical of other Paediatric Cardiac Surgery units in England at the time.'

Bristol was an entirely avoidable tragedy. Had the surgeons taken note of Ernest Codman, concentrated on the simpler operations they could do well and referred the difficult operations to other units with the appropriate expertise, there would have been no scandal. Complex paediatric heart surgery needs specialist paediatric heart surgeons, and Bristol didn't have one. They had two adult surgeons in their mid-fifties trying to do the really hard stuff with staff shortages and shocking facilities. They should have recognised their own limitations during surgery, and instigated an inquiry after one unexpected death, not thirty-five. And when they refused to stop, the Department of Health and Royal College of Surgeons should have stepped in to stop them.

Private Eye didn't stop the surgeons either, but it certainly had an effect. In 1992, no UK surgeons were releasing their figures to the public and I guess that having them released for you in a satirical magazine, especially when they were this bad, might just piss you off rather than make you stop and think. Once you're in siege-mentality mode, it can be hard to break out of it and my exposure may just have contributed to that.

The public inquiry didn't report until 2001, which tells you how accountable the NHS was at that time, but they performed an impressive audit trail of the *Eye* articles which at least proved that everyone in authority knew about Bristol, and they might even have done something about it had the president of the Royal College of Surgeons not gone on holiday and missed a vital meeting at the Department of Health. The figures for Bristol stuck out like a sore thumb as far back as 1989, but while they remained unpublished, they could be hidden and parents were left in the dark. One *Eye*-reading couple did at least write to health secretary Virginia Bottomley to ask for her advice.

25 May 1992

> Dear Mrs Bottomley,
> We were disturbed to read in a recent edition of *Private Eye*, a report about the paediatric cardiology unit at Bristol. The column implies that a child undergoing surgery in Bristol stood less chance of surviving than in other parts of the country. Our child is due to have an operation in Bristol in the very near future, to try to alleviate a congenital heart defect. We have been warned that there is a one-in-four chance of failure and we are now concerned to know if the risk may be reduced if the operation were to take place elsewhere.

Just one month later, Ms J Binding, from Corporate Affairs at the NHS Management Executive at the Department of Health bounced the letter back to John Roylance, the chief executive at Bristol:

22 June 1992

> Dear Dr Roylance,
> The attached correspondence has just (sic) been received. It raises matters which can best be dealt

with by your Trust. I would be grateful if you could look into the matter and reply directly to [the parents]. I do not need to have a copy of your reply at this stage but I may need to ask for one later.

Clearly Mrs Bottomley and the NHS Management Executive weren't keen to get involved. The next reaction to the *Eye* came from Sir Keith Ross, an eminent retired cardiac surgeon from Southampton who had set up a Working Party to report to the Department of Health on units carrying out child heart surgery. He should have known what the Bristol figures were, so I was puzzled by the letter he wrote to senior Bristol heart surgeon, James Wisheart:

7 July 1992

Dear James,
I am writing to you in some distress because I have just been told of a comment about Bristol paediatric cardiac surgery, supposedly by someone who could only have been me by inference, in *Private Eye*. Please accept my complete and unqualified denial of any such comment – not only have I not discussed your unit with anyone outside the Working Party, I can honestly say I have no knowledge of your results. I can only assume that some malicious person who knows I sit on the Working Party has, for some reason best known to himself, seen fit to ascribe this comment to me. As always in this situation, there is nothing I can do except acquire an even deeper hatred of the behaviour of the press.
With kind regards,
Keith

28

Ross later admitted that he knew Bristol's overall figures were poor compared to other units, but didn't have a breakdown of individual operations. I was hoping the *Eye* might spur him into investigating, but he and Wisheart were old friends who had worked together. As Ross told the inquiry: 'James made a good impression as a conscientious and meticulous young surgeon ... we altogether enjoyed a satisfactory personal relationship and when my time finished on the Council of the British Heart Foundation, I had no hesitation in recommending him as my successor.' Ross could have been, but clearly wasn't, the man to support an investigation at Bristol.

However, the *Eye* nearly managed to get a result thanks to a letter from Dr John Zorab, a consultant anaesthetist and medical director at Frenchay Hospital in Bristol. He wrote to Sir Terence English, another eminent cardiac surgeon, immediate past-president of the Royal College of Surgeons and a member of the Department of Health's Advisory Group, which oversaw the provision and funding of paediatric cardiac surgery services.

15 July 1992

> Dear Terence,
> Sometime last Autumn, I made one or two efforts to get to see you in order to discuss the delicate and serious problem of mortality and morbidity following paediatric cardiac surgery in Bristol. Great anxieties were being expressed by some of my colleagues at the Royal Infirmary. In the event, I never made contact and the matter passed from the forefront of my mind.
>
> Matters have come to a head once again and the enclosed piece from *Private Eye*, whilst possibly having some inaccuracies, quotes some statistics

that have been confirmed elsewhere. One of the newer consultant cardiac anaesthetists feels that the mortality rate is too distressing to be tolerated and is job-hunting elsewhere.

Whether the *Eye* is correct in saying that the matter has already been drawn to the attention of the College and the NHS Management Executive, I do not know. There is, however, a widespread feeling that the situation is well-recognised but being ignored – possibly because no-one knows how to tackle it.

Yours sincerely

John

Again, this letter shouldn't have been too much of a surprise. Back in 1989, Ross's Working Party reported to the Advisory Group that Bristol had a higher mortality rate than the other units. The medical secretary of the Advisory Group, Dr Norman Halliday, told the inquiry that when Bristol was given the Department of Health's seal of approval to operate on babies and children in 1984, it 'did not actually shine like a star' and 'performance was not on a par with other units.'

The hope was that performance would somehow improve. It didn't. In October 1986, Professor Andrew Henderson of the University of Wales distributed a letter at a meeting of South Glamorgan Health Authority stating 'it is no secret that their [Bristol's] paediatric cardiac surgery service is regarded as being at the bottom of the UK league for quality.' Dr Halliday was informed but felt he could not take the case further as no supporting evidence was attached.

In 1989, Halliday received the Working Party report outlining poor outcomes in Bristol and, in 1990, he visited the unit and noted 'sub-optimal' results, attributed to the low volume of work. In February 1992, Dr Halliday was handed

Bristol's very poor 1991 figures but he 'didn't have the machinery to analyse the data'.

Bristol was a well-known and long-standing problem that should have been sorted out long before *Private Eye* put it in the public domain in 1992. Dr Zorab's letter convinced Sir Terence English to 'revisit the 1991 figures on mortality'. He now realised that the Bristol unit stood out as far worse than anywhere else, even though the Working Party had recommended that it should carry on. In his reply to Zorab, English wrote:

27 July 1992

> Dear John
> . . . I will make a full response when I return from holiday in mid-August. Suffice it to say at this stage Bristol is not included in the paediatric cardiac surgical units recommended by the Royal College of Surgeons for continued designation for supra-regional funding. The Working Party report will be considered by the Advisory Group on 28th July.
> Yours sincerely
> Terence

So although Ross's Working Party had recommended that Bristol be allowed to continue despite the bad results, the Advisory Group was going to overrule and recommend funding be withdrawn, which would stop the surgeons operating. Alas, English was off on holiday and would miss the vital meeting, but he agreed this plan of action with Professor David Hamilton, a colleague from the Royal College of Surgeons who would be attending. And he wrote a letter to Professor Norman Browse, who had just replaced him as president of the Royal College of Surgeons:

24 July 1992

Dear Norman,

... In the [Working Party] report, which is to be considered on 28th July, Bristol was included as one of the centres for designation. However, it is clear from a review of the report that their mortality statistics, both for the infant age group and the older age group, are worse than any other centre. David Hamilton agrees that sufficient attention was not paid to this by his Working Party. We agreed, therefore, that to allow Bristol to go forward with support from the College might jeopardise designation of the whole service and, with David's agreement, I have spoken to Norman Halliday who will inform the Advisory Group on Tuesday, 28th that the College does not support the inclusion of Bristol; I am sure this is the right action.

Yours sincerely
Terence

Private Eye, thanks to John Zorab, had got the Royal College of Surgeons to see sense. Or it might have done had Sir Terence not been in Pakistan. When he returned, there was a letter waiting for him from Professor David Hamilton:

3 August 1992

Dear Terence,
I hope that you had a highly successful trip to and safe journey back from Pakistan, and are refreshed after a demanding but successful term as President. Following our telephone conversations of

Thursday evening, July 23rd, and Friday afternoon, 24th, I was not entirely happy about our agreement to take action over the Working Party's report. On reflection, I realised a possible specific source of breach of confidentiality which could arise and a further feeling that the de-designation of one of the units would probably leak out in the course of time.

Also, the members of the Working Party were unanimous in their findings and gave considerable thought to their recommendations. Like you, I was unable to contact Keith Ross, but did so early on Monday morning, the 27th, after he had returned home from holiday. He was equally concerned that we had changed the report and suggested on reflection that we should both speak with Norman Halliday to reverse the decision and the instruction that you had given him.

. . . The Working Party could be requested by the Advisory Group to reconsider the mortality figures of specific units (or unit) and possibly to amend its findings. This appealed to me as a far safer course of action.

Yours sincerely

David

Safer for whom? The Advisory Group refused to take action against Bristol to protect babies from unnecessary death because the data from all units had been collected in confidence and if Bristol was 'struck off', it would be obvious that it was the one with the really bad results that stuck out like a sore thumb (and which everyone knew was Bristol anyway). Such was the mindset in 1992. And, as Keith Ross pointed out, there was an unfortunate holiday clash:

When David Hamilton phoned me, I had just returned from Scotland and had no idea of the events leading up to the telephone call ... I must have agreed with his concern regarding the Working Party's conclusions being altered but there was no way I could have talked to Terence English as he was either in or on his way to Pakistan. ... In fact, the convergence of so many factors at the end of July 1992, which included Dr Zorab's letter, a new President of the Royal College of Surgeons and the absence of Sir Terence English (and for that matter myself) from the Advisory Group meeting was a historical disaster.

Ross's Working Party never revisited Bristol's mortality figures. English told the inquiry that he specifically raised them with Dr Halliday, but Halliday disputed this. The matter was never even raised at any future Advisory Group meeting, even though they were both members. The high death rates were not investigated and Bristol continued unchecked until the death of Joshua Loveday three years later.

By 1995, the surgeons had supposedly agreed to stop the more complex operations until a specialist paediatric cardiac surgeon was appointed. But they pressed ahead with Joshua's surgery despite opposition from anaesthetic staff, other surgeons and the Department of Health. Joshua died, the shit hit the fan and the rest of the media finally cottoned on. Even the General Medical Council woke up and instigated one of the biggest arse-covering operations in the history of medicine.

Why did no-one step in earlier? As Bristol inquiry chairman Ian Kennedy observed with some anger: 'One of the features of our taking evidence is that no matter whom we have spoken to – whether it be a health authority, a trust, a royal college and now a department [of health] – they have always found someone else responsible.' His comments were in response to the evidence of Sir Graham Hart, a permanent secretary at the Department of Health until 1997. In Sir Graham's view: 'Ministers who are politicians should not be involved in the clinical treatment of patients,' and there was a 'deeply rooted reserve' against the department becoming involved in monitoring clinical performance.

Doctors can't have it all their own way. If they want to regulate themselves and not have politicians interfering in clinical matters, they have to be open about their results. Publication of outcomes is essential to maintain trust, as is sound statistical analysis to identify a 'significant outlier' that needs swift investigation. And politicians, civil servants and managers shouldn't just plough money into a failing service in the vain hope it will get better.

Kennedy later referred to the process of designating which centres should perform child heart surgery as having 'all the qualities of a Greek tragedy. . . . Bristol was frankly not up to the task. . . . There is real room for doubt as to whether open heart surgery on the under-1s should have been designated in Bristol.' The inquiry tried very hard not to blame anyone but concluded that 'in certain respects, when concerns were raised, in the roles they then occupied, Dr Halliday and Sir Terence English should have behaved differently.'

When I gave evidence to the inquiry, I was vaguely threatened with a custodial sentence for not revealing all my sources. (I realised then that I probably should have brought a lawyer along.) I then received a warning letter saying that the inquiry might criticise me for raising concerns in *Private Eye* rather than 'the usual channels' but they backed off, presumably when they realised how ineffectual the Royal College of Surgeons and the Department of Health were.

The General Medical Council (motto: 'Protecting patients, guiding doctors') wasn't much use either. Having failed to protect any babies, they jumped in before the public inquiry to save face and pin the disaster on three doctors: the two surgeons, James Wisheart and Janardan Dhasmana, and the hospital chief executive John Roylance, who was also a doctor.

Roger Henderson, QC for the GMC, left little room for doubt: 'Mr Wisheart should have realised by 1993 that the mortality of up to 54% associated with the operations he carried out to correct atrioventricular septal defects – compared with the national average of 13.9% – was comparatively disastrous.' But the GMC didn't define statistically what it meant by 'comparatively disastrous'. Twice as bad as the national average? Three times? Four times? Unless you set this safety standard, there is no automatic trigger to tell surgeons to stop operating and start investigating.

Wisheart had voluntarily stopped operating before the GMC inquiry. An external assessment of his adult surgery between January 1993 and September 1995 found that his 30-day death rate for lower-risk arterial bypass operations was 12.2% versus an average of other consultants of 2.6%. When it came to all coronary artery bypass operations, Wisheart's death rates were 13.4%, compared to the average of 4.1%. He was described by the auditors as 'a higher risk surgeon' with a performance that 'appeared to be significantly poorer than the others.' He'd gone off the boil all round, hardly surprising given the stress he was under.

The GMC found that the two surgeons 'had continued to perform certain operations despite growing concerns about poor mortality figures. They did not adequately establish the causes of those results. One of them misled parents about likely outcomes. And the then chief executive failed to take action when colleagues voiced anxieties.' In 1998, the GMC struck off Wisheart (who had retired) and Roylance, and suspended Dhasmana (whose adult figures were good) from carrying out child heart surgery for three years.

The GMC is very good at punishing doctors long after the event, but its claim to protect patients has never quite stacked up. Until he retired, Dr Michael O'Donnell was the longest-serving member of the GMC and chairman of its professional standards committee. In a statement to the inquiry, he wrote: 'Over lunch at a GMC council or committee meeting, I'd raised the subject of what seemed to be happening in Bristol, almost certainly prompted by what I'd read in *Private Eye*. Though one or two of the people I discussed it with seemed concerned, the general reaction was one of intense apathy.'

Five years later, when the GMC was forced into action, O'Donnell 'got a number of phone calls from doctors in and around Bristol who hadn't realised I was no longer on the GMC, wanting me to know what a good chap Wisheart was and wondering if I could "do anything" to get the charges dropped. One of the callers assured me, rather alarmingly, that someone in the past had managed to "do something" about another case.'

O'Donnell also revealed details of two GMC health screeners 'who had to decide if a doctor's ability to practise might be impaired by any illness or alcohol dependency. The pair were known to have "drinking problems" and yet were allowed to remain in office. . . . I raised my concern about the first screener with the then president. The problem with the second was so widely known that the secretariat tried to ensure that alcohol was not available at midday during meetings of the Health Committee.'

The journalist in me is very good at exposing scandals in black and white in under 800 words, but it took a public inquiry lasting two and a half years, with evidence from 577 witnesses and 900,000 pages of documents to make sense of what happened in Bristol in the broader context of a ludicrously underfunded and overburdened health service. The report of the inquiry, chaired by Ian Kennedy, is one of the wisest documents ever written about the NHS, and had its 198 recommendations been followed, the NHS would be a safe place to be sick in and I wouldn't be writing this book now. You can still access the report at www.bristol-inquiry.org.uk

The report points out that 'the story of the paediatric cardiac surgical service at Bristol is not an account of bad people. Nor is it an account of people who did not care, nor of people who wilfully harmed patients.' This was why they were so hard to stop. They weren't depressed or alcoholic or psychotic, they were workaholics. They should have stopped, but their unit would have lost funding and prestige. So they carried on.

The surgeons' supporters, and there are many, point out that their commitment and dedication were beyond doubt, the majority of their operations went well and that the biggest factor in their downfall was the understaffing and inadequate facilities they had to contend with. While these were indeed appalling, the inquiry stressed: 'It is crucial to make clear the following. The inadequacy of resources for paediatric cardiac surgery at Bristol was typical of the NHS as a whole. From this, it follows that whatever went wrong in Bristol was not caused by lack of resources. Other centres laboured under the same or similar difficulties. For example, the shortage of qualified nurses and cardiologists was a national phenomenon, affecting all centres. We therefore emphasise the point again that, while under-funding blighted the NHS as a whole, it does not alone provide the explanation for what went wrong at Bristol.'

The inquiry noted that the Bristol team showed a lack of insight and teamwork, poor communication and flawed behaviour. Hardly a recipe for safety. To perform paediatric cardiac surgery successfully, you need a functional team at the top of its game. I doubt my *Private Eye* articles helped teamwork or morale, not least because they spread mistrust: 'Which of you bastards has been speaking to the press?'

When I gave evidence to the inquiry, I said that the Bristol surgeons were fall guys for a much wider problem in the NHS – a complete lack of accountability. All doctors were pretty much free to do what they wanted, guided only by their clinical judgement, and that's a pretty dodgy compass. I didn't quote Codman, but I called for all surgical teams to have their outcomes measured, adjusted for risk and published. If the NHS provided a truly good service, this would restore trust and confidence. If it didn't, we needed to act.

Heart surgeons were first to grab the nettle. Since publication, mortality rates are continuing to fall and there's no evidence that sicker patients are being denied surgery. But the rest of the NHS remains a big black hole that we're only slowly shining a torch into now. As Kennedy pointed out on July 18, 2001: 'Even today, it is still not possible to say, categorically, that events similar to those which happened in Bristol could not happen again in the UK; indeed are not happening at this moment.' And we still don't know, seven years later.

More Scandals on the Bottomley Watch

PRIVATE EYE

16 February 1994
The inadequate resuscitation facilities in Liverpool hospitals first highlighted by sacked nursing student Kenneth MacDonald in 1991 have been further exposed in the *British Medical Journal*. MacDonald complained that whilst working at Walton and Fazakerley hospitals, two patients were left to die when the cardiac arrest ('crash') team should have been called. The *BMJ* study of 297 patients at Fazakerley Hospital found that nearly a third of these were deemed not for resuscitation (NFR) by the medical staff (usually in the absence of a consultant) and in only a third of these cases had the

prognosis been discussed with relatives. Nurses and doctors were sometimes unable to agree on whether to resuscitate, with the result that for five patients, the nurse didn't call the crash team even though the doctor wanted them to. MacDonald believes that such cases could be tantamount to manslaughter and has asked the Mersey constabulary to investigate.

20 February 1994
Mrs Bottomley's dubious defence of community psychiatric care in the wake of the Clunis Report centred on a small increase in the number of community psychiatric nurses (CPNs). At present, there are 5,000 such nurses and six million people with mental health problems. For schizophrenia alone, only one person in five has access to a CPN and there are likely to be at least a hundred patients as disturbed as Christopher Clunis, who stabbed Jonathan Zito to death at Finsbury Park tube in 1992, walking around London at the moment. Ironically, it was the public outcry over lack of community supervision of such disturbed patients which initially led to the construction of long-stay psychiatric hospitals, many of which have now been closed (and sold off for housing). The report has asked for an urgent increase in the number of medium-secure beds in south-east London, where 45% of GPs have no access to mental health professionals whatsoever, and more general psychiatric beds in inner London.

How should doctors deal with violent patients? Stoke GP Dr Kauser Jafri has admitted to carrying an imitation .38 Smith and Wesson revolver in his doctor's bag for the last seventeen years for 'confidence and personal safety'. When faced with 'a drunk drug addict who was menacing and swore', Dr Jafri found it particularly useful: 'I tried to appear calm but a chill ran down my spine. "Let me just examine you" I said very deliberately as I opened my bag. I took out my stethoscope slowly giving him the chance to see my revolver. The effect was stunning. His whole demeanour changed and I was able to send him away with just one day's supply of drugs.'

24 March 1994

Last year, anaesthetist Behrooz Irani was struck off after he switched off alarms on anaesthetic equipment at Humberside's Castle Hill Hospital and left a patient, who turned blue and had no heart beat for seven minutes, in a permanent vegetative state. Now the chairman of the anaesthetic division of East Yorkshire NHS Trust has been found guilty of serious professional misconduct by the GMC for failing to relieve Irani of his duties despite a number of warnings from senior operating department assistants.

Irani previously worked at Hull Royal Infirmary, where consultant surgeon Mr Alan Wilkinson had to administer artificial respiration to bring one of his patients round after the anaesthetic. Mr Wilkinson told the GMC hearing that 'the man was not safe' but added: 'In Hull we do not have consultant anaesthetists growing on trees. I didn't make a formal complaint because it was either him or nobody. We are constantly having to do that because we are so understaffed.' After leaving Yorkshire, Dr Irani worked as a locum in Chepstow, Gwent, until he was sacked after leaving a patient, whose oxygen level was dangerously low, to make a telephone call.

10 June 1994

Junior doctor Alan Massie died in January after working a continuous 86-hour shift in obstetrics and gynaecology at Warrington District General Hospital, just three years after the BMA and Mrs Bottomley decided that such stressful, unrelenting jobs should convert to a shift system, with no doctor working a longer stint than eight hours. The tribute to Dr Massie from the nursing staff at his funeral read: 'Always smiling, always tired, always hungry.'

18 August 1994

All is not well at Royal Oldham Hospital. Ten junior doctors have written to trust chairman Mary Firth claiming that 'gross understaffing' on the medical wards has led to 'dangerously inadequate levels of care.' Patients have to wait hours to be assessed by a doctor and the trust had to close to emergencies on several occasions in June and July. The elderly ward is staffed at half the recommended level, causing 'an impossible situation for the remaining on-call staff. The attention given to individual patients is desperately lacking on a day-to-day basis, and their admission stay is undoubtedly prolonged beyond what is necessary.' As Ms Firth observed: 'This is just a little blip.'

25 March 1995

'Institutions', claimed Bertrand Russell, 'are to be judged by the good or harm they do to individuals.' The latest Office of Population Censuses and Surveys figures show that nurses top the league for female suicides, with 153 ending it all between 1990 and 1992. The second most at-risk group is female doctors and indeed seven of the top ten high-risk groups are professions related to medicine.

6 July 1995

Mrs Bottomley's last-gasp announcement as health secretary that the intake to medical schools is to be increased by 10% by the year 2000 may have come too late to solve the medical manpower crisis. It costs the taxpayer £192,000 to train a medical graduate, but up to a quarter of newly qualified doctors now give up or disappear abroad. Many parts of the NHS only function thanks to the efforts of overseas doctors, who occupy 26% of the training grades. In some specialties such as anaesthetics, psychiatry, paediatrics and general practice, there are often no applicants for jobs advertised in the

British Medical Journal. Increasing the student intake is unlikely to have any effect if the working conditions remain so poor. As one of this year's Birmingham graduates put it: 'When I first went on the wards in 1992, all the junior doctors told me to give up now and all the consultants said it would be alright in the end. Now everyone's telling me to get out.'

Just as alarming is the national shortage of consultants. There are 150 national consultant vacancies in anaesthetics alone, with trusts resorting to head-hunting, poaching, overseas recruitment and inflated salaries to fill posts. Dr Julia Moore, clinical director of anaesthetics at Merseyside's Wirral Trust, claims trusts are no longer advertising vacancies in the UK because they know there'll be no replies. As health minister Gerry Malone put it: 'I disagree with the words "manpower crisis".'

STEPHEN DORRELL
July 1995–May 1997

Stephen Dorrell is probably best known for wearing a chunky-knit, cuddle-me sweater to one of William Hague's informal love-ins, but his time as health secretary was marked by the fag end of the Major government and the emergence of two scandals, BSE and Bristol. No wonder he looked like a man tortured by irritable bowel syndrome.

In March 1996, Dorrell told the Commons that it was likely that the first ten cases of a rare brain disease called new variant CJD were due to exposure to beef products contaminated with BSE. Measures to prevent transmission of BSE to humans had been introduced back in 1988–89, so this shouldn't have been a news story. Bad luck then that every paper led with 'Mad Cow Killer' headlines and everyone stopped eating beef apart from John Gummer, the agriculture minister, who force-fed his daughter a burger for the camera. No-one would import British beef, farmers were rushed into the mass slaughter and burning of cherished herds and £3 billion went in compensation for what was essentially a non-scare. As Dorrell told Radio 4: 'It's not the cows that are mad, it's the public.' Clearly he was courting the dead cow vote.

Bristol emerged as a public scandal in 1995, and Dorrell ordered an inquiry. But it was left to Frank Dobson to decide whether to make it public, or to keep hiding the bad stuff.

PRIVATE EYE
New Wine in Old Bottles

4 August 1995

This October heralds the start of a huge country wide change in undergraduate medical education, with the introduction of the GMC's 'new' curriculum. Instead of cramming two hundred medical students into a sweaty lecture theatre or sending them off to cut up dead humans and live domestic mammals, they will now have their values explored in small focus groups before being dispatched into the community to learn about real life. Or so the theory goes.

The changes have met with a lot of resistance, principally from those who stand to lose financially. It costs the taxpayer £34,000 a year to train a medical student, so a medical school with a thousand students rakes in £34 million a year. Only a fraction of this has ever gone on teaching, with professors preferring to use the money to tart up their departments and conduct research. A typical surgical unit in a teaching hospital might receive £4 million a year in teaching money, and in return will allow a few students a week to tag onto the end of a ward round or hang on the end of a surgical instrument. Disciplines such as anatomy, physiology and biochemistry stand to lose most as the factual content of the course is slashed and replaced by subjects such as 'How We Learn' and 'Real People, Real Problems'.

The biggest problem facing medical education is not, however, the course content but the 'see one, do one, teach one' ethos of British medicine. Very few medical teachers are taught to teach, preferring to rely on their innate abilities. This, coupled with the patronage system that prevents juniors from complaining, has allowed many eminent consultants to humiliate their students over the years without fear of reprisal.

One consultant general surgeon at Birmingham's Selly Oak

Hospital prides himself on his amusing banter over the operating table. As a female student put it: 'First he asked me if I was from the home counties. When I said yes, he started calling me Tinkerbell and said I looked the sort of girl who'd had a horse between my legs. Then he asked me if I'd lost my virginity up against the wall of a horsebox while my mother was outside watching a gymkhana. The surgical registrar and the other theatre staff started laughing too. It was like being in a monkey house. At the end, he asked me if I minded him being sexist in theatre: "Women like to know what men want." Then he made a hole in the gall-bladder and said: "Look what you've made me do."'

Another consultant surgeon at the Queen Elizabeth Hospital was recently forced to apologise in writing to a female student after saying, 'You must have felt testicles before. Haven't you got a boyfriend?' Changing the curriculum without changing the attitudes of the staff could be disastrous. As Stanislaw Lec put it: 'If you give a cannibal a fork, is it progress?'

Pill Scare

20 October 1995
'I am acutely aware that this new information will worry women, and impose a substantial burden on doctors and pharmacists.' So said Professor M D Rawlins, chairman of the Government's Committee on the Safety of Medicines (CSM), in his letter informing every GP in the UK that seven of the most popular oral contraceptives should be abandoned for women with risk factors for venous thrombo-embolism such as obesity, varicose veins or a previous history of thrombosis of any cause. 'Other women', concludes Rawlins, 'should continue to take them only if they are intolerant of other oral contraceptives and prepared to accept the increased risk of thrombo-embolism.'

Unfortunately, this information reached me twenty-four hours after it hit the press and not in time to reassure a surgery full of women, most of whom had no notion of the absolute and relative risk. The overall odds of a non-smoking under-35-year-old woman dying as a result of taking the pill are 1 in 77,000. For a pill-taking smoker under the age of 35, the odds are 1 in 10,000. The non-smoker is thirteen times more likely to die while driving a car, six times more likely to die as a result of pregnancy and two and a half times more likely to die in a household accident than from taking the pill. Two themes emerge: death on the pill is rare and if you want to reduce your risk, stopping smoking is far more important than which pill you take.

As for the risk of vein clots, these in themselves are inconvenient but only dangerous if the clot breaks off and bungs up the lungs. Venous thrombosis occurs in 1 in 10,000 non-pill-takers every year. Pill-takers were thought to have a 2 in 10,000 risk, but Professor Rawlins seems to be suggesting that those taking any of the magnificent seven may have a 3 in 10,000 risk. As 70% of the women in our practice are on these 'harmful' contraceptives, I wanted more evidence than a flimsy circular from the CSM before embarking on the wholesale disruption of their family planning.

This would not seem unreasonable, since this Government is constantly exhorting the value of evidence-based medicine, a founding principle of which is that grass-roots doctors should not accept the judgement of detached academics, but evaluate the evidence at first hand from the original scientific papers. This is even more important when an author of one of the papers, Professor Walter Spitzer, strongly disagrees with the CSM's interpretation. Earlier this year, the Government tried to blacklist these newer contraceptives on financial grounds, so I was naturally anxious that this might be part of the hidden agenda. Fortunately, Professor Rawlins' letter ended: 'If you require any further information, please call.'

When I phoned to ask for copies of the three unpublished papers on which this advice is based, I was told: 'You are not allowed to see the evidence.' When I pointed out that this was for my personal analysis of the validity and reliability of the studies in question, the phone went dead. Why should the trials be kept secret from doctors? At present, all I have is dozens of worried women and two Sainsbury's bags full of returned Marvelon and Femodene. Any offers?

Unkind Cuts

6 December 1995

'It is pointless to perform major surgery on patients who are physiologically compromised unless there are facilities for those patients to recover post-operatively.' So said the fourth annual *Independent National Enquiry into Perioperative Deaths in England, Wales and Northern Ireland*. Of the doctors surveyed, 81% had access to intensive care beds but only 21% had access to high-dependency units, which closely monitor patients who are still too sick to return to a general ward.

Lowlights of the 19,816 deaths that occurred within 30 days of operation include a 70-year-old man who underwent emergency surgery to repair a strangulated hernia, only to find the recovery room was closed for the night (he died 15 hours later) and a 54-year-old man who was admitted to a university hospital with a head injury. There were no neurosurgery beds available and the CT scanner was out of commission, delaying the diagnosis. When the need to operate was spotted, the two specialists were busy opening someone else's skull, resulting in a 5-hour delay. He died 16 days later.

A Junior Doctor Writes

18 January 1996

Dear Sir

I am a house officer at Wansbeck General Hospital, an institution that has featured several times in your column. Despite having been a doctor for only five months, I consider myself hardened, cynical and brutalised. I have seen my interests and hobbies decimated and have lost touch with friends because of my job. In February, I move to a trust in Sunderland, where my contract has been vetted and declared 'totally unacceptable' by the BMA's industrial relations officer. In August, I will join the hordes of junior doctors fleeing Britain to New Zealand, Australia and South Africa because I cannot envisage doing 3–4 more years as a senior house officer, working for these disgusting institutions.

At Wansbeck, a trust millions in debt, we admitted medical emergencies to surgical wards almost every day over Christmas and New Year. This is distressing for the nurses, who are not used to this type of patient, and bad for patients themselves who can easily be forgotten. On one weekday following New Year, 18 of 21 emergency medical admissions between 17.00 and 09.00 went to surgical wards, and a ward had to be re-opened to cope with demand. At the moment, the plan is to cut the number of medical beds despite year-round bed-occupancy rates well over 90%. The only thing that has made the job bearable is the 'in the trenches' camaraderie amongst junior doctors.

If you use any of the above, please don't mention my name. As you know, medicine is a patronage system and seems very sinister from where I am.

A Patient Writes

13 February 1996

Dear Sir,

Being disabled in my late forties, I wear a calliper on my leg and cannot walk far because I suffer from angina and asthma. Last Tuesday, I was admitted to the East Surrey Hospital at 9pm with an asthma attack. I was told that there were no beds available and that I would have to stay in the casualty department until one became free. After four hours on a hard trolley, I had an X-ray taken before being put to sleep in a very noisy plaster room. Next day, I thought I would be transferred to a ward. Not so. In fact, I was kept in the casualty department for three days and three nights, after which I was completely exhausted.

There was nowhere to wash, except in a small hand bowl, and just one toilet nearby. There wasn't enough bed linen and twice I had my pillow taken away from me when I left it. The noise was unbearable and the food arrived at 6pm and 8am, with nothing in-between. One night I was woken by a nurse trying to take my oxygen supply for another patient, and another nurse remonstrating with him saying that I needed it.

It's not the fault of the medical and nursing staff that these appalling conditions prevail. Indeed I feel sorry for them as all the time they were rushed off their feet. Their morale is at its absolute lowest. The nursing staff suggested that if I was not happy I should write and complain, as their grievances are constantly ignored and they can do little or nothing to get improvements. Who is to blame for all this? Is it just a lack of funds or what? It certainly needs sorting out.

Yours sincerely,
Mrs Gwen B Ross

A Relative Writes

6 June 1996

My father reached Princess Alexandra Hospital (Harlow) by emergency ambulance at 12.45pm on February 12, following a phone call from his GP stipulating that hospital admission was essential. On arrival, a notice board in reception informed us that we could expect a 3-hour wait due to staff sickness. My father was wheeled on an ambulance trolley into a draughty corridor where my mother and I waited with him for two hours. During that time, a nurse took his pulse, temperature and blood pressure, and gave him an oxygen mask. However, despite his obviously deteriorating condition and our repeated request for further examination, none was forthcoming. At 2.45pm he was allocated a cubicle, but was not seen by a doctor until 6.45pm.

The doctor who eventually examined him said that he was extremely dehydrated, which came as no great surprise as my mother and I had repeatedly expressed our concern to several members of staff that he was unable to tolerate any food or drink for over two days. However, we were told that no food or drink could be administered prior to being seen by a doctor. Before any action was taken to rehydrate him, he had to endure a series of X-rays when he was clearly in severe distress and lapsing into unconsciousness. By the time a drip bag was produced at 7.15pm, it took ten minutes to locate a drip stand. His oxygen tank was replaced, but only after I pointed out that it was empty. The soap dispenser in the cubicle was empty and no pillow could be found to support his head.

At 10pm, the doctor we had previously seen informed us that a line would have to be inserted into my father's neck, and politely asked us to wait outside. Several doctors came and emerged shortly afterwards to tell us he required urgent renal dialysis. My father was transferred to the Royal London Hospital at 11pm after a further delay due to a non-starting ambulance and a failure to locate some jump leads. On arrival at the Royal London, he was immediately allocated a bed and dialysis was commenced. This was unsuccessful and he was again transferred, to the intensive care unit at Bart's Hospital, where he died without regaining consciousness.

My father suffered from a serious illness, but had he received prompt medical treatment he would have at least been able to say his last goodbyes to us. Our devastation and heartbreak would have been terrible in any event without this additional burden to bear. I have since obtained a copy of the Patients' Charter for the people of North Essex which states that patients can expect to be treated with 'dignity and privacy' and that the 'care environment will be quiet, warm and comfortable'. This was not the case. He also has 'a right to emergency medical treatment at any time in the A&E department' but no timescales are mentioned, which merely compounds my cynicism.

A Consultant Writes

30 June 1996
Letter from Dr J E Carty, consultant rheumatologist, Lincoln and Louth NHS trust

For some time there has been a developing inequality between the services we provide to (non-fundholding) GPs through the Lincolnshire health contract and those to GP fundholders. Whilst there is no difference in the treatment and clinical decisions we make about patients, the access time for surgery is now a cause for great concern. There were many worries when GP fundholding was established that there would be a two-tier system: that certainly exists and in fact we have a several-tier system, with some fundholders seeking non-urgent surgery within three months and most within the 9–12 months range. For non-fundholders, we only guarantee the Patients' Charter Standards of 15 months for hips, knees and cataracts, and 18 months for everything else.

To give an example, one of my colleagues has undertaken the sterilisation and removal of a coil for a fundholder patient who has been waiting no more than 6 weeks, but is not able to give treatment to a Lincolnshire health patient with a fibroid uterus and debilitating heavy periods until mid-1997. This is unsettling and causing professional concern. We wish to treat patients on the basis of clinical need and not by virtue of the accident of where they live and the practice they are signed up with. This is supposed to be a National Health Service funded by universal taxation.

A Manager Writes

Letter from Tracey Baggott, contracts manager for GP Fundholders at Southampton University Hospitals NHS Trust

Due to financial pressures, some health authorities have had to take the difficult decision to impose service restrictions within their contracts and allow the waiting times for their residents to move out beyond previous targets. In order to manage this difficult situation, I am writing to request that all general practitioners could indicate on their referral letters to this Trust whether they are fundholders or not, for example by putting GPFH under their signature. This would enable the Trust to prioritise patients, if applicable. This will also help avoid consultants being placed in an awkward position whereby they are unsure whether the patient belongs to a fundholding practice or is the responsibility of the health authority, and will allow the consultant to give his patient a more accurate estimate of their expected waiting time.

Dr Phil's Notes

After eleven years in power, we're all keen to give Labour a good kicking, but looking back on my time under the Tories shows how they failed to make the NHS safer or sort out variable standards in care (and access to it). They introduced a management structure obsessed with money and efficiency without any responsibility for safety and quality. In such a system, danger thrived.

BLAME LABOUR
1997–

BLAME LABOUR

In opposition, Labour got NHS staff on their side by deriding the Tories' internal market as iniquitous and wasteful, and pledging to dismantle it. In office, they embraced it wholeheartedly, but not before ditching GP fundholding. The scheme was clearly unfair in that patients from these practices got quicker care than those from practices that were too small to qualify, or had ideological objections. But the danger of enforced equality is that it breeds mediocrity. The NHS needs room for innovation, even if some patients get it before others. Many fundholding GPs were both innovative and wise, grouping together to provide a whole range of services closer to patients' homes. They could also bypass hospitals if they had concerns about the quality and safety of care.

Eleven years of Labour and a vast sum of public money later, the English NHS is stuck with a market for healthcare. Our only hope is to keep it local and build on what we've got, rather than selling off NHS services to overseas corporations. If Labour had developed fundholding, allowing GP practices to pool their budgets and develop partnerships with managers, hospital staff, IT experts, social services, local businesses and charities, it would have been a far faster route to the integrated, localised, safer NHS that we're still grasping at.

The Bristol scandal, and much of Shipman, happened on the Tories' watch. But it was left to Labour to decide how to deal with the fallout. Would they see it as an opportunity to embrace quality and safety in the NHS? Or would they use it as a stick to beat and control doctors, and drive through their secret privatisation agenda?

FRANK DOBSON
May 1997–October 1999

Dobson was a surprise replacement for Chris Smith, who was publicly against the private finance initiative and made a rash pledge to save Bart's Hospital. Dobson was hardly 'new' Labour, promising to abolish the internal market but then not being allowed to. Gordon Brown did, however, honour his commitment to stick to Tory spending plans, and so much of Dobson's term of office was taken up with fire-fighting stories of scandalous waits and lack of resources.

Dobson was committed to improving quality and reducing inequality, and was persuaded by lobbying parents to hold a public inquiry into the Bristol heart scandal (but not until after the GMC had tried to save its skin first). Dobson generally got on well with everyone, until he took his shoes off. But he pissed off a few doctors by saying on *Newsnight* that he wouldn't let Janardan Dhasmana, the Bristol heart surgeon suspended from operating on children, operate on him. Blair saw him as a night watchman, to lull the electorate and Old Labour into a false sense of security before unleashing Alan Milburn.

Dobson was set up to fail, sent in to bat for the NHS without a helmet, box or pads. Or a bat. With no extra money, he just had to take the flak for the 'epidemic of hospitals short of beds, doctors hunting for beds and patients turned away' that he'd railed about in opposition. Dobson has since found a second wind as backbench opposition to the commercialisation of the NHS, where he speaks with passion and zeal but very little influence.

PRIVATE EYE
Misinformed Consent

20 June 1997

A study of unsupervised surgical training published in the *British Medical Journal*[1] has confirmed what many doctors, and very few patients, suspect: two-thirds of all operations performed by surgeons-in-training are unassisted. Senior house officers are left alone to do their first salivary-gland excisions, hernia repairs and stomach, spleen and gall bladder removals with senior 'support' not even present in the hospital. One rung up the ladder, surgical registrars are doing complex and life-threatening surgery of the liver, gall bladder and pancreas, often in emergency situations. Emergency bowel resections, leaking aortic aneurysms and kidney transplants are all done for the first time unsupervised. The list for head-and-neck surgeons is so unsettling as to be almost unprintable (e.g. radical neck dissection), and even consultants had to perform operations they hadn't witnessed before.

The analysis of all this has focused on the shambles of medical training, brought about by a combination of professional arrogance, dereliction of duty and, most pertinently, because we have fewer doctors per head of population than most other countries in Western Europe. As one consultant put it: 'If every surgeon had to prove competence prior to performing any procedure, the NHS would collapse overnight.'

Another conclusion is that many operations performed in the UK could be subject to legal action. Doctors have a duty to gain informed consent from patients prior to any procedure. According to the GMC: 'every patient has the right to make his or her own decision regarding medical treatment and care, and

---

[1] *British Medical Journal* 21 June 1997.

in order to make that decision is entitled to have full information regarding the material risks.' What risk could be more material than a junior surgeon performing your major operation for the first time unsupervised? And yet, NHS patients are seldom given information as to the identity of their surgeon, and never whether he or she has proven competence for the operation.

Informed consent has always been a myth. Often consent is left to the junior house officer, who may not have seen or heard of the operation. As a house officer, I consented someone for a choledochoduodenostomy and I'm still not sure what it is. The GMC suggests that patients should only be consented for operations by someone who is competent to perform it. It would help if the person performing the operation could prove his or her competence too, or at least be closely supervised by someone who could. Alas, neither of these goals is achievable with the current level of staffing in the NHS. Some surgeons argue that most trainees performing solo operations for the first time achieve satisfactory results, and that should be enough to reassure the public. However, far too many cockups still occur and, for the relatives left behind, discovering the truth is a painful and prolonged business.

If doctors are to continue with the responsibility of regulating themselves, then the least they could do is follow the American example, where surgeons publish audits of their work that are freely available to the public. A few fiddle their figures to make it look like they're doing harder operations (thus making their results appear better than expected) but generally it works well. For trainee surgeons, figures can be grouped with the consultants who are responsible for their training.

Some surgeons argue that British people are too dim to interpret the results and incapable of making allowances for variations in case-mix between surgeons. Those who only operate on low-risk patients will, almost invariably, achieve better results than those who include high-risk (i.e. very unwell) patients. However, it is quite possible to produce two columns of, say, mortality figures, one which lists the predicted mortality for a particular operation based on the case-mix and average UK results, and another that lists the actual mortality of a particular surgical team. And it doesn't take a genius to spot a team that is way below average.

If surgeons are as competent as they would have us believe, then they have nothing to fear from public audit. If not, then health secretary Frank Dobson will have to find a lot more money for surgical training.

Waiting for Sight

15 August 1997
In the last week, I've seen two patients waiting over eighteen months for cataract operations. Their vision has now deteriorated to such an extent that one is effectively housebound and the other regularly scalds herself with the kettle and is covered in bruises from multiple falls. The operation they both require is extremely successful and quick. It can be done as a day case and is therefore not affected by bed blocking from the increase in emergency admissions. The NHS hospital they have been referred to has a full quota of eye surgeons and offers private cataract operations with a nine-day wait. Those who can't afford to pay are waiting seventy-times as long to be treated in the same NHS hospital by the same surgeon using the same equipment. Frank Dobson's pledge to end two-tierism in the NHS is already looking mighty thin.

Labour may blame the previous Government for inheriting the largest ever rise in waiting lists (up 13%, with 47,000 waiting over a year), but it has also inherited an NHS with more money and more surgeons than ever before. The problem lies in what the surgeons actually do. In 1995 the Audit Commission discovered that an average full-time NHS surgeon does just 3–6 hours at an NHS operating table per week. This compares with 20 hours a week in most other EU countries. Indeed, if NHS surgeons operated on NHS patients for just fifteen hours a week, then no-one would have to wait more than six days for an operation. The NHS would become just as fast and remain a lot safer and cheaper than the private sector, removing the need for the current, grossly iniquitous system. So why hasn't it?

Many surgeons are desperate to be given more NHS operating time, as witnessed by the number who put in extra hours in aid of the Conservatives' waiting-list initiative. Outrageous waits of six years or more have all but disappeared, and the 250,000 patients waiting more than a year for surgery in 1989 were reduced to 4,756 by September 1996. Some surgeons claimed that this political expediency had allowed those waiting longer for routine operations to leapfrog over those waiting a shorter time for urgent surgery, but there is little hard evidence for this. The average NHS wait during this time rose slightly from 34 to 42 days, but the scheme was a temporary success. Alas, when the Conservatives stood back and fed the NHS to the internal market, the log-jam quickly reappeared.

Surgeons themselves are not without blame. They control the waiting lists and those with a keen interest in private practice are less enthusiastic about reducing NHS waits. NHS surgeons at present only have to work a maximum of 3.5 days a week, leaving them plenty of time to pursue other interests. The private system in the UK allows insurance companies to write policies that cherry-pick easy acute cases in healthier people, leaving the NHS to provide for the chronic, difficult cases and the very sick. In addition, the NHS has for years acted as a free safety net to bail out private hospital disasters. The response has been not to improve the free service so as to make private care unnecessary, but to invest in additional NHS paybeds to try to undercut private hospitals.

At present, the NHS employs a large number of consultant surgeons at £50–£70,000 a year (plus pension and perks) who are given the ridiculous operating resources of half a day a week. Teaching, research and administration take up more time, and outpatient clinics can be one never-ending cattle market. But there's also some paid thumb-twiddling and absconding to private competitors. A better solution for surgeons who want to commit to the NHS would be to offer them full operating and audit facilities throughout the year, and pay them to be genuinely full-time (i.e. no private work). Their work could then be targeted at areas of greatest need – like giving old people the gift of sight.

Still Waiting

29 August 1997

My views on waiting lists provoked a balanced response from the medical hierarchy. The suggestion that NHS surgeons are not used in the most efficient way and that some favour private work over NHS commitments was dismissed as 'nonsense' and 'rubbish' by Dr Peter Hawker, deputy chairman of the BMA's Central Consultants and Specialists Committee: 'Everyone knows that the problem is funding.' Even a spokesman from the Royal College of Surgeons was nudged into a response: 'These are unsubstantiated claims . . .'.

Whilst underfunding is clearly the biggest problem facing the NHS, the claim that private practice is detrimental to the NHS is hardly unsubstantiated. In 1995, Dr John Yates of Birmingham University published *Private Eye, Heart and Hip*, which cited clear evidence that waiting list reductions in the UK have in part been hampered by some consultants spending an inappropriate amount of time with private patients. The response from the BMA was predictable – one representative made a vitriolic personal attack on Yates's motives and political views in a radio interview – but the response from grass-roots surgeons was divided. One wrote of his embarrassment at the failure of the profession to tackle abuses, another – on a maximum part-time NHS contract – boasted that four-fifths of his operating was private.

Protectors of the private faith have always argued that it benefits the NHS – that patients who pay for treatment aren't added to NHS lists – but Yates's research in Birmingham showed that consultants cannot be in two places at once and when they try to serve two masters, it is the NHS that suffers. Not that this evidence was easy to come by. He was repeatedly thwarted in his attempts to discover the truth but, with the help of observation by private detectives, managed to compile a formidably detailed dossier of the detrimental effect of private medicine on NHS waits.

Did it do any good? When he presented *prima facie* evidence of abuse at a Birmingham hospital to the regional health authority, they distorted it so much as to conclude no problem existed. The Conservative Government decided to gloss over it too, leaving an angry but persistent Dr Yates searching for more evidence to encourage the NHS to change. He has been joined by Professor Donald Light from Manchester University, who wrote in 12 July's *BMJ*: 'The (current) arrangement provides strong incentives to minimise (i.e. ration) operations for NHS patients and use the NHS as an operating base for maximising private work ... I have been told by consultants that some surgeons walk out with NHS X-rays for their private patients under their arm. This is stealing. If a cook walked out with a ham, she or he would be arrested. Some surgeons work out deals with GPs to take care of their NHS patients promptly, if the GPs will steer patients who can pay over to their private practice. Some surgeons are said to manipulate their waiting lists and what they tell a given patient in order to get patients with money to go private. I am told the distorting effect of these "sweetheart" contracts lead the minority who exploit them to believe that politicians and NHS patients should feel grateful for whatever work they do for the NHS.'

The abusers are very much in the minority and it is far more common to find that NHS surgeons work for more hours than they are paid for. However, for the BMA and Royal College of Surgeons to pretend that none of their flock work the system for pecuniary incentives truly is nonsense, rubbish and unsubstantiated.

Addicted Doctors

19 December 1997
Spare a thought this Christmas for addicted doctors. There are thirteen thousand of us in the UK still practising the noble art whilst dependent on alcohol or drugs – an unbelievable statistic if it didn't come from the British Medical Association. The BMA is trying to tackle the problem through a 24-hour stress line launched in April 1996. In the first year, 3,300 calls were received, 57% from women doctors, who make up a third of the workforce. A third of the calls dealt with emotional problems (anxiety, stress, depression), a quarter complained about work practices, but very few admitted to an addiction problem. And even fewer were prepared to whistle-blow on a colleague.

The ability of doctors to hide their addictions stems from a combination of intelligence, professional status, peer loyalty and lack of insight. Those who are aware they have a problem are also mindful of coming forward because, according to Dr Clive Froggat, 'there is no effective support system available. Your whole livelihood is threatened and there is little effort put into rehabilitation. So an awful lot of sick doctors are just allowed to practise by their colleagues.'

Froggat has been very public about his addiction since he was exposed in 1995. He started with cannabis as a medical student and progressed to cocaine and heroin in 1989. He got the former on the black market and the latter out of his bag, and for years hid the problem from his wife and partners until a Cheltenham pharmacist became 'deeply suspicious' about his prescribing habits. A month later, there was a very public dawn raid on his house.

Dr Ian Joiner is a recovering alcoholic who still practises as a GP. He has a drinking history spanning 35 years from medical school, peaking at four bottles of gin a week and four drink-driving offences. Dr Joiner was placed under psychiatric supervision for seven years by the GMC and now runs the Addicted Physicians Programme from his front room in Farnham, Surrey: 'Recently I spoke to a cardiac surgeon who was drinking half a bottle of vodka a day so he could steady his hands before an operation. He was unable to take my advice and he's still out there.'

Dr Joiner set up his service in 1995, funded entirely by donations from users, because he was disillusioned by the help offered by the medical establishment. The occupational health service in the NHS is scandalously poor, and it's left to a patchy 'three wise men' procedure in hospital and on Local Medical Committees to sort out problem doctors and protect the public. The National Counselling Service for Sick Doctors offers an informal route to psychiatric services which, in the current climate of the NHS, often fail to provide the necessary supervision to rehabilitate doctors.

The General Medical Council has ultimate responsibility to

protect patients but currently just 140 out of the 13,000 addicts are practising under the GMC's supervision. The GMC's view is that, whilst recognising that it only sees the tip of the iceberg, the local procedures work well to sort out addicted doctors and it's not something the public should worry about. Clive Froggat takes a different view: 'If there are 13,000 addicted doctors making 2,000 vital clinical decisions each year, that's 26 million vital decisions each year made by addicts.' Cheers!

It's hard to find evidence of wholesale patient harm at the hands of addicted doctors, largely because no-one picks up doctors' mistakes. Earlier this year, a fatal-accident inquiry at which it was alleged a consultant surgeon operated under the influence of alcohol led to calls to breathalyse surgeons. Pilots and train drivers have to do it, and doctors may follow suit.

The BMA has set up an action group in Scotland for problem drinkers, but seems to have conceded that what's needed – a humane working environment and a good occupational health service – may never happen. Last month, the BMA gave a huge vote of confidence to the NHS by sending its members details of BUPA personal healthcare with preferential discounts. So now we can all get pissed in private. Merry Christmas.

Pain Special

30 December 1997

If you had crippling pain following an illness, operation or accident, you might expect someone to sort it out. Soon. Certainly, we have the knowledge and the technology. As Dr Douglas Justins, a consultant anaesthetist and pain-management specialist at London's St Thomas's Hospital puts it: 'It's 151 years since the first anaesthetic was given in Britain and in this day and age it's totally unacceptable for anyone still to be suffering acute pain anywhere in a hospital.' Alas, an Audit Commission Report, *Anaesthesia under Examination*, has found that only 57% of hospitals have acute pain-control teams which have been proven to reduce and often eliminate suffering, and that the amount of pain you suffer can depend on which hospital the ambulance drops you off at.

All this prompted Leo Strunin, president of the Royal College of Anaesthetists and a consultant at the Royal London Hospital, to accuse NHS trusts of failing to take patients' suffering seriously: 'Many do not see it as a quality issue. The funds and leadership just aren't there to provide proper pain relief in hospital.' How comforting. Earlier last year, another report found that children, from neonates on special care upwards, suffered unnecessary pain and that new approaches such as needle-free analgesia aren't filtering through. In adults, half of all cancer patients and a third of cardiac patients suffer unnecessary pain. Although there has been a 41% increase in the number of consultant anaesthetists over the last ten years, this has been well outstripped by demand and 13% of posts are vacant. Many trusts have barely enough anaesthetists to put people to sleep, let alone administer epidurals to labouring women or run pain clinics.

At undergraduate level, training in pain management is often pitiful, and many health professionals qualify with quaintly stoical views about pain and a reticence to use opioid pain-killers. Morphine is a brilliant painkiller and has been used for centuries, and yet many doctors either refuse to give it or don't give enough for fear of overdosing or causing addiction. 'The reluctance to prescribe morphine is a long-standing problem based on tradition, misconceptions, misinformation and a lack of education,' says Justins. 'It is perceived as a very dangerous drug.' In fact, even when patients are on large doses to control their pain, the chances of becoming a drug addict are 'infinitesimally small'. Over time, the body does become tolerant to the drug and larger doses are needed, but these don't result in overdose. It's far more likely for pain to kick in because a doctor is reluctant to increase the dose.

The best pain relief we have remains misunderstood and underused, as roofer Rod Buck can testify: 'I fell 30 feet off a roof and landed on my back. I broke most of my ribs and the broken ends penetrated the lungs. . . . In intensive care, the pain was overwhelming. It was out of this world, it actually paralysed you, you couldn't move, all your muscles clamped up and you were absolutely frozen rigid.'

After two weeks of pain and much forceful complaining, Rod got what he needed: 'I was rescued by an anaesthetic consultant who had a special interest in pain management and prescribed morphine for me. But once I got on the general wards, I was aware of a subtle disapproval on the part of many of the staff of me being on morphine, rather as if I was a sort of an alcoholic or child molester, certainly a person of weak moral fibre, because I was needing to take this stuff.

'I think my experience was unusual because I demanded and got adequate analgesia. I think a lot of people give up in the face of determined opposition of the nursing and junior medical staff.'

Take a tip from Rod. If you suffer excruciating pain in 1998, ask for some morphine. And a pain specialist. Happy New Year.

Cervical Screening is Hard

12 February 1998

The cervical screening fiasco in Kent and Canterbury (eight women dead and 250,000 smears to be rechecked) may not be the only one. The interpretation of slides of cervical smears is not clear-cut or simple, and a decade ago standards were not in place in many labs where poorly paid, overworked screeners had five minutes to interpret what were often very complex cell patterns. As a result, there are potentially twenty or more labs around the country where, if you rigorously examined the work they were doing eight or ten years ago, it would be no different to Kent and Canterbury.

Given the current level of media and legal interest in this topic, it is likely that these centres will be exposed over the next few years. Although surgeons can bury their mistakes, pathologists (and radiologists) leave concrete records of each test, which years later can be given to an expert with hours to spend, knowing that the patient subsequently developed a problem.

Screeners remain overworked and under enormous time pressure today, but all labs now operate double-checks and use safety-net procedures, and overall the incidence of cervical cancer deaths has fallen. Many people mistakenly believe that with immaculate screening, cervical cancer can be eradicated completely. This has never been true, given the unpredictability of some forms of the cancer. For every cancer detected, one will escape detection even with the best screening.

A far greater problem is that just as most labs are getting it right, the adverse press from the consequences of yesterday's low standards is making it extremely difficult to recruit high-quality technicians. Mr Dobson may throw money at the problem but if no-one wants to do the job, the screening programme will be stuffed. Then see what happens to cervical cancer rates.

Cleft Lip and Palate Surgery

26 February 1998

Last November on *Trust Me, I'm a Doctor* (BBC2), I exposed the dismal state of cleft lip and palate repair in the UK, with large numbers of centres doing relatively few operations with poor cosmetic results. A North West of England audit had found that 48% of children require major and often multiple reconstructive surgery, Royal College of Surgeons guidelines were being flouted, and a petty turf war was being fought out by plastic surgeons and maxillo-facial surgeons to the detriment of patients. Now, four months later, the Clinical Standards Advisory Group of the Department of Health has agreed.

After investigating 297 children aged five, and 277 aged twelve, who had all undergone cleft repair in Britain, they found that 40% had poor dental bite, less than a third had a good lip appearance at the age of twelve and under half could speak with normal intelligibility at that age. The CSAG stated that of the 57 centres carrying out the operation, only six to eight provided good-to-excellent care and the overall results were five to twelve times poorer than in the six European centres examined. And the key factors causing poor training and poor results were 'specialists' doing only one or two operations a year and 'competition between plastic and maxillo-facial surgeons'.

It is now almost six years since the *Eye* published the equally unimpressive audit figures for paediatric cardiac surgery at the Bristol Royal Infirmary and highlighted the need for surgical teams not just to audit their work but to act on the results, retiring gracefully from operations which may be beyond them. This latest report found that not only are many surgeons continuing to perform operations they are not competent to do, but they are failing to keep adequate records or perform proper audit.

Only in the area of alveolar bone grafting is there enough information to compare the two specialties and the results are not pretty. 50% of cases carried out by plastic surgeons failed, compared to 32% done by maxillo-facial surgeons. A further factor in this gross incompetence was the desire of hospital managers to keep operations in-house and cheap rather than refer to a more expensive super-specialist centre which may do 50 successful operations a year using highly trained teams.

The false economy and inhumanity of the former approach is illustrated by Dr Symon Whyte, an anaesthetist who had to undergo nine major corrective operations in his childhood because the first repair was not done properly. One operation stuck in his mind: 'It involved breaking the upper jaw on both sides, advancing the jaw so that the bite came into a normal line, taking some bone from my left hip, and grafting that into the gap they'd created in the fracture site. They then welded the whole lot into place with plates so that it was fixed and rigid and the bones could grow together again.' Seven hours in theatre, 24 hours in intensive care, wires and tubes everywhere . . .

Viagra etc.

6 May 1998

British men itching to get their hands on Viagra (sildenafil) – the impotence pill not yet available on the NHS – are trying their luck in Harley Street. However, they should be very wary of the mark-up. Some private clinics have an abysmal record of ripping desperate men off, and prey on the assumption that they will be too embarrassed to question the fee. Many sufferers prefer to answer anonymous private ads in the press than confront their GP – whose knowledge and attitudes may in any case be unhelpful. An Impotence Association Survey found that half of those men who do see a GP come away dissatisfied and 23% get no treatment at all.

If they do, the commonest prescribed impotence drug in the UK is Caverject (alprostadil), which works in a similar manner to Viagra by relaxing smooth muscle and increasing penile blood flow – but has to be given as a shot in the shaft (not too painful though, I'm told). Alas, impotent men who decide to go private commonly end up paying over £1,000 for a short consultation (worth £60), a few blood tests (worth £100 at most), a trial intra-penile injection of Caverject (£7) and, if it works, a few doses to be getting along with (£30).

A much better and cheaper impotence service is available in parts of the NHS, but you may have to persevere to find it. Some GPs are happy to initiate treatment but others prefer to refer to a hospital clinic, usually run by a urologist or a specialist nurse. Caverject is available on the NHS or, if you prefer, the same drug can be given intra-urethrally (down the end of the penis) in pellet form. This is amusingly known as MUSE. If either suits, you'll be given a small supply and referred back to your GP, who must then decide how much to shell out for your sex life. There is great variability here. As Sister Nolly Biggins, an impotence specialist at Doncaster Royal Infirmary, puts it: 'The good GPs recognise the distress and marital breakdown that impotence can cause and will prescribe enough of the drug for sex twice a week. But I have known male GPs who'll only dish out enough for once a month. I mean, what do they think their knob's for – stirring the tea?'

Viagra, Caverject and Muse don't work for everyone and are not without side-effects. Vacuum pumps have been around for years. They're very effective, and have very few side-effects, other than a very cold penis. But for some ludicrous reason they are not available on the NHS. As Sister Biggins explains: 'They're very useful for diabetic men, half of whom become impotent and many don't want to take any more drugs. But because the pumps aren't prescribable, I've had to buy some using charitable donations and share them out amongst the patients.' At £200 each, they're not cheap but they recoup the cost of drug treatment in a few months.

Some men who can't afford them buy cheap penis pump enlargers from sex shops or mail ads. 'They're a disaster,' says Sister Biggins. 'They don't work properly and they usually give you a tight plastic ring to slip over the base of the penis to maintain the erection. Often, the ring's so tight that it won't come off and you have to go to casualty to get it cut off.' You have been warned. Always use a penile ring with handles attached.

Colorectal Cancer

20 May 1998

In 1997, the NHS executive published the research evidence for 'improving outcomes in colorectal cancer'. This is the second biggest cancer killer, causing 17,000 deaths a year in England and Wales. It gets more common with age and often presents with bleeding from the rectum or a change of bowel habit.

The survey found large variations in the methods used and success rates for surgery, and concluded that 'surgery for rectal cancer should be concentrated in the hands of surgeons who can demonstrate good results, particularly in terms of low recurrence rates. Surgeons should monitor their performance by working closely with histopathologists.' But only 5% of them do and the rest really haven't got a clue how they're doing.

Even when a surgeon meticulously audits his work and proves that a new technique can bring substantial benefits, it can take fifteen years for these to become widely used. Bill Heald, a Basingstoke surgeon, has pioneered the technique of total mesorectal excision (TME) which involves meticulous removal of the tissues lying circumferentially around the rectum, rather than the traditional process of removing a tumour longitudinally. Recurrence rates, colostomy usage and death are markedly lower in his patients compared to those elsewhere in the UK, and although no randomised controlled trial has been done, population studies in Scandinavia, Holland and Germany are strongly reinforcing this finding. Heald has revolutionised rectal cancer care outside the UK.

The fact that Heald's genius has been embraced by our European partners but largely ignored in the UK says a lot about the way we practise. Surgical training has not in the past allowed the specialisation to learn new skills such as TME, preferring to produce general surgeons who can do a bit of everything. Some can, but others are getting alarmingly high recurrence rates for the cancer and recurrence nearly always means death.

Back in 1986, Heald published his own recurrence rates of 2–6% compared to the national average of 35%. His colostomy rates are 15%, compared to the average of 45%, and by preserving the nerves of sexual function, his impotence rate is also a third that of those using traditional surgery. Indeed, there is more variability in the outcomes for rectal cancer surgery than for any other cancer, so it's vital you get a specialist team that publishes its results.

Eye Plug

3 July 1998
'The role of non-executive members of healthcare trusts has become an issue; their absence from the Bristol story is remarkable, especially given that stories in the satirical magazine *Private Eye* put the issue on the public agenda (a fact that should surely have alerted everyone that there was enough

dissent among staff to persuade someone to leak information to the press).' So observed Rudolf Klein, professor of social policy at Bath University in the *British Medical Journal* (June 6, 1998, p. 1742).

The baton for sorting out this mess will soon be passed to Professor Ian Kennedy, who is to chair the public inquiry. In the meantime, it's worth pointing out that the new paediatric cardiac surgery team in Bristol have mortality rates lower than the national average. For the first time in six years, I'd allow my own children to be operated on there.

A Surgeon's Lot

17 July 1998

At London's Royal Brompton Hospital, cardiothoracic surgeons are effectively on call 24 hours a day, every day. As one put it: 'The policy here is that if a patient that you operated on develops a problem, you are expected to sort it out even if you aren't officially on duty. So you have to carry a pager with you all the time, and be prepared to come back to theatre.' Quite why the surgeons are so reluctant to sort out each other's complications is unclear – perhaps they don't wish to contaminate each other's league tables – but committing to round-the-clock cover means never touching a drop of alcohol, just in case they're called in. What a life.

Although individual surgeons will not be identified when Frank Dobson publishes the rates of post-operative death and other selected complications, surgical units will be named and consultants are worried that they may be tainted by association. The least they can hope for is that a statistical adjustment is made to favour the units who do the hardest operations on the sickest patients. Poor results will be blamed on the consultants, even if the problem operations are done by junior staff, since they are responsible for the training. As one consultant told me: 'We're resigned to the fact that league tables will be here to stay after Bristol, but a lot of us are worried. Even if they're accurate, everyone has a bad year or a bit of bad luck or a poor batch of junior staff every now and then. In the past, we've managed to sort it out in private – but once it's public, a single blip could stuff your private work for good.'

Aortic Aneurysms and Biliary Atresia

31 July 1998

An aortic aneurysm is an abnormal bulging of the major vessel that carries blood out of the heart. 3% of men over 50 have one, usually without any symptoms, and at least a third of these will go on to rupture. This is bad news. Symptoms include severe abdominal pain, often radiating to the back or groins, and collapse. The emergency surgery involves clamping the aorta above the leak and inserting a Dacron graft. Without treatment, the death rate is 100%. With treatment, the death rate depends on how quickly it is picked up – large ruptures at home have a 90% death rate, in hospital the average survival is 50%.

However, a much better outcome can be achieved by screening. With ultrasound, most of the aneurysms can be picked up and operated on before they rupture. When this policy to screen men over 60 was introduced in Chichester, the death rate from ruptured aneurysms fell to zero (i.e. there weren't any) and the death rate from the elective operations was just 1%. In two-thirds of the cases, the aneurysms might not have ruptured but the pick-up rate was far higher than, say, cervical screening and comparatively many more lives were saved. And although expensive in terms of the initial outlay for screening and the elective operating, the patients didn't require the prolonged intensive care that those having emergency surgery often need. This can lead to a miserable prolonged death from kidney failure and infection.

After the elective operation, the men are then brought back to the mortality rate of their peers (i.e. they live as long as men who don't have aneurysms), giving them up to twenty years extra of high-quality living. So presumably every major centre around the country is offering screening? Alas no. Men who've worked hard and paid tax all their lives are still thought of as low-priority patients, it seems. The cynical view is that it is much cheaper to let them collapse at home and die. As one consultant put it: 'We're probably losing 6,000 men a year through not screening men over 50. Compare that with cervical screening, where we screen all women aged 20 to 65 and save a thousand lives a year.' Without screening, your best bet for survival is to call an emergency ambulance if you get the above symptoms and go straight to hospital.

At the other end of life, my top tip is to take jaundice in babies seriously. Any baby that is still yellow at two to three weeks needs to be assessed. The cause is usually breast-feeding, but biliary atresia, a congenital malformation that prevents bile drainage, must be excluded. And yes, there's a scandal here too. If children are identified early (within six weeks), often they can have a complex operation called a Kasai procedure that takes up to five hours but can improve drainage through the biliary tract. At best, this can completely obviate the need for a liver transplant or at least postpone it for many years. At worst, it does nothing, other than subject a very young baby to life-threatening surgery.

Because the condition is rare, only 50 such operations are carried out in the UK each year. So you'd think they're all done in two or three highly specialised centres which do enough of the procedures to ensure they're good at them. Unbelievably, there are fifteen centres doing the operation, with many carrying out just one or two a year. King's Hospital London and

Birmingham are the centres of excellence, doing most of the operations and clearly they should be doing them all – their success rates are double those of the dabblers. So if your child is offered this operation at another centre, insist on going to King's or Birmingham.

More Biliary Atresia

27 August 1998

The Kasai operation is a complex procedure used to correct biliary atresia, a congenital malformation that prevents bile drainage, and two factors determine its success: (a) the speed with which the diagnosis is made and (b) the skill of the surgical team. At best, the children remain jaundice-free for many years and may never need a liver transplant. At worst, the operation fails and the baby needs a transplant to survive in the next year or two. So the stakes are high.

Back in 1985, the *British Medical Journal* published a survey of the results of this treatment conducted between 1980 and 1982.[1] Ninety-five children had the Kasai operation. They were treated at sixteen different centres by at least sixteen different surgeons, and success was measured according to whether the children were free of jaundice from 10 months to 3.5 years. Good results were clearly related to the number of cases operated on in each centre. Only 11% of children treated in centres dealing with one case a year were free of jaundice compared with 29% at centres treating two to five cases a year and 45% at King's College Hospital, London – the only centre to treat more than five cases a year.

[1] McClement J, Howard E, Mowat A. Results of surgical treatment for extrahepatic biliary atresia in United Kingdom 1980–2. *British Medical Journal* 2 February 1985; 290: 345–7.

The paper deduced that this alarming variability in results was 'probably' down to 'the experience of the surgeon and the standard of care'. It concluded that the outlook for these children would be improved if 'treatment was concentrated in a few centres, in each of which the vast majority of operations are done by one surgeon'. Thirteen years later, you'd imagine it was all sorted out. Dream on. The survey for 1993–95 found that fifteen centres were still doing the Kasai operation and although the overall success rates have improved, the same depressing variability exists.

The average success rates for the two units doing more than five operations a year (King's and Birmingham Children's) is 62%, those doing two to five is 50% and those doing one a year is 17%. Based on this information, I recommended that children should only be referred to King's or Birmingham. This provoked a prompt response from Mark Stringer, a consultant paediatric surgeon at Leeds General Infirmary, whose own figures are comparable to the best. So Leeds can be added to the recommended list, but I wouldn't go to units that do one operation a year. As Mr Stringer puts it: 'We need to prevent surgeons carrying out this operation on rare occasions and the British Association of Paediatric Surgeons has been taking steps to achieve this.' It's now just thirteen years since their last survey proposed to do exactly that. But hey, it's only eight-week-old babies we're dealing with.

And what of the parents? The downfall of the surgeons in Bristol was not their poor performance *per se*, but that they had quoted parents national survival rates for operations when their own figures were far worse. Are parents of children with biliary atresia treated at the 'one a year' centres being told the local success rate is 17%, compared with 62% elsewhere? I suspect not.

On the Nose

11 September 1998

A patient recently turned up to ear, nose and throat outpatients at Southampton University Hospitals NHS trust and was turned away for being a year early. He hadn't spotted that the waiting time for a routine appointment (i.e. the time taken to see a doctor even before you go on the waiting list) is 60 weeks. This is clearly unacceptable, but hardly surprising when you consider that there are more ENT consultants in New York State than the whole of the UK and clinics are already ludicrously busy. One junior ENT surgeon in Leicester regularly sees more than 30 patients in a three-hour outpatient clinic and his record is 44. This works out at four minutes per patient, including turnaround time, when the recommended appointment time for good-quality practice is fifteen minutes. Clinics become cattle markets and everyone ends up dissatisfied.

The obvious solution is to train more junior staff and create more consultant posts for them to go to. Alas, this can meet barriers from managers ('too expensive') and some existing consultants who don't want anyone cutting into their lucrative private work. In Southampton, two of the ENT specialists have vetoed another consultant appointment and opted instead for an associate specialist. Associate specialists cost less than a consultant but very few are accredited for their training, some have repeatedly failed membership or fellowship of their royal college, and the ones I've met are deeply unhappy and disillusioned with their lot. They can never become consultants but they're allowed to do a lot of the consultant's work, usually unsupervised. This is hardly a guarantee of the quality service Frank Dobson bangs on about, and yet the *BMJ* job section is full of adverts for associate specialists.

In the short term, Dobson is trying to solve the problem of long waiting lists by paying consultants private-size fees to operate on NHS patients in private hospitals at weekends. For example, the orthopaedic consultants in Southampton have received £2.5 million to get their lists down. This strategy – also used unsuccessfully by the Tories – comes on the back of a report by the charity Action for Victims of Medical Accidents, which has found that a disproportionate number of the claims it deals with are coming out of the private sector. Key factors are the lack of both emergency equipment and medical expertise. Private hospitals are not the places to be in an emergency.

A Surgeon Responds

24 September 1998

The *Eye*'s exposure of variable success rates for surgery in infants with biliary atresia has provoked an interesting response from surgeon Andrew J McIrvine:

'You have fallen into the fallacy that large numbers are a necessity for excellence. The statistical fact is that you cannot interpret the results from the centres with low numbers. In simple terms, a one-a-year centre can only have either 100% success or 100% failure. Putting all these centres together and giving a figure of 17% is simply unfair.

'This problem holds true for many other surgical procedures. Carotid endarterectomy [scooping out muck in the carotid artery to prevent a stroke] should be another one ripe for investigation and audit. The Vascular Surgical Society did such an audit but was unable to relate frequency of operation to success rate. Although you quote one paper, there is very little evidence of this linkage. The data to support super-specialisation is very thin, it may be that really extreme specialisation makes you more dangerous again as you cannot deal with anything outside your very narrow field. As we have relatively few surgeons in this country we just cannot afford to be so specialised.

'As an individual surgeon, it is even more difficult. Say when you start your consultant career you have a series of bad results. How do you know whether it is you, or just statistical bad luck? The overall stroke rate associated with carotid surgery is usually quoted at 4%. If this was your first 4 cases, it could be surgical incompetence, if it was the last 4 of 100 it would just be regarded as luck, but in both series it could be down to chance. Lord Brock is famously quoted as killing his first ten mitral valvotomies. Numerous other operations started with high failure rates. For how long are surgeons meant to hold their nerve while attempting new procedures and developments?

'It must have taken considerable nerve to try the Kasai operation at all. It does not make logical sense just to stitch a bit of bowel to a liver with no bile ducts and hope it will drain but it does work, up to 62% of the time in the best hands. You can be sure the early results were not this good. It is very easy to knock those surgeons with poor results, but by definition as biological creatures some surgeons will be better than others, so will their supporting teams, physicians, anaesthetists, nurses etc. Success or failure is likely to be multi-factorial. If we witch-hunt all surgeons to have figures only as good as "the best" the result will be that the majority of surgeons will just stop doing any risky surgery. The ultimate question, then, is will society benefit overall? This would only be the case if you believe that the general standard of surgery is so low that stopping surgeons operating will save lives. (Of course my anaesthetist wife supports this point of view!)'

This is all fascinating stuff, but the question remains – should surgeons be prevented from doing once-a-year complex operations if facilities are available in centres of excellence which do more of the procedures and get much better results?

Statistical proof of any surgical team's competence is notoriously difficult to find as the numbers are usually small and there are in any case no defined minimal standards. But there is evidence for more common procedures that more is better. For example, centres doing more than 100–200 Coronary Artery Bypass Grafts a year have a lower in-hospital death rate.[1] A lot of surgery is about making a judgement without statistical proof, and if I had to choose between a high- or a low-volume centre, I'd go high every time.

Shouldering the Blame

22 October 1998
The *Eye*'s exposure of the trend for NHS trusts to appoint cheaper, less-qualified associate specialists rather than new consultants has rung bells with a junior obstetrician who wishes to remain nameless. 'Appointing consultants rather than associate specialists is a far better way of meeting clinical needs and safeguarding standards. But managers want to save money and existing consultants don't want to share their private practice or scarce NHS resources (secretaries, offices etc.).

'There will soon be 200 fully qualified, UK trained and accredited specialists in obstetrics and gynaecology without a consultant post. Meanwhile, concerns about safety and the lack of experience of obstetricians in operating theatres and labour wards persist.'

The potential danger of this lack of experience was recently highlighted by David Wrede, a senior registrar in obstetrics who is now working in Australia because he couldn't get a

---

[1] Snowden et al. The Relationship Between Hospital Volume and Health Care Outcomes, *CRD Report 8*. NHS Centre for Reviews and Dissemination, York, 1997.

consultant post here: 'In the current (UK) system, the first time you see an obstetric emergency like shoulder dystocia (when the baby's shoulders get stuck) is at night as a green registrar with the consultant at home and unable to assist. If you are lucky, all goes well and you go off duty shaken enough to read everything you can about shoulder dystocia for the next time. If not, the experience haunts you both personally and at the next audit meeting, where you are not usually severely criticised for acting where you had no proven competency.

'After five years as a specialist registrar, you may have seen enough cases to feel comfortable managing the condition and then get a consultant post. The irony is that you then do your on-call at home and may never be directly involved in a case again. For the highest quality of care and training in acute specialties, fully trained specialists will have to be resident on-call.' Mr Wrede's forthright views may not have helped him get a consultant post, but he is adamant about the need for a consultant-led service despite the professional resistance: 'One consultant leader was heard to say, "Consultants resident on-call? Over my dead body!" Yet if doctors profess to uphold the highest standards of acute care, whose dead bodies are we talking about?'

If Frank Dobson is genuine in his desire for a quality service, he has to fund sufficient consultant expansion in all specialties to allow them to lead the service and supervise junior doctors around the clock. The plan to recruit more medical students is laudable, but they won't be consultants for twenty years and then only if there are sufficient posts created for them to go to. Some will doubtless help the manpower crisis in general practice, but without consultant expansion, the benefits for hospitals will be negligible.

Blind Amniocentesis

19 November 1998

If you were pregnant, would you let an obstetrician stick a needle into your uterus without knowing where the baby is? It happens every day in the UK. Amniocentesis involves drawing off fluid from around the baby in the womb to diagnose conditions such as Down syndrome. It's usually performed at sixteen weeks and parents are told that the risk of causing miscarriage is between 0.5% and 1%. However, in some hands, the risk may be much higher. An unpublished audit at a centre in Wales found a miscarriage rate of 4%, eight times worse than the best centres. Why?

A successful amniocentesis depends on the needle reaching the amniotic fluid in the womb without hitting the baby. For over fifteen years, ultrasound equipment has allowed continuous monitoring so that the needle tip is always in view during the procedure, as well as the placenta and the baby (which has a habit of moving around). It requires training and considerable skill to operate the ultrasound equipment and guide the needle at the same time and, as you'd expect in a service as patchy as the NHS, some obstetricians (both junior and senior) don't have it. But they do amniocentesis anyway.

How? They do the ultrasound first, find out where the baby is, put the scanner down, pick up the needle and hope that the baby doesn't move. But often it does. And even if you manage to avoid the baby, you may hit the placenta which can have equally catastrophic effects. Bad amniocentesis can not only cause miscarriage, but there's increasing evidence it could also lead to brain damage in surviving infants.

If amniocentesis is done blind, the only way of knowing you're in the right spot is if the syringe is filled with clear amniotic fluid. If it's filled with blood, you've bodged up, but you get rid of it quickly, hope the parents don't notice and have another go. This is clearly unacceptable practice, but it wasn't until 1996 that the Royal College of Obstetricians and Gynaecologists got round to issuing guidelines, stating that amniocentesis must be performed under continuous ultrasound with the tip of the needle always in view.

Alas, Royal Colleges carry very little clout and some obstetricians just carry on doing it the old way. Eric Jauniaux, a foetal medicine expert at University College Hospital sees a woman a week who has had a failed amniocentesis: 'In most of the cases they tell me that there wasn't any ultrasound guidance at the time of the procedure.'

As with most of medicine, training is poor and there's very little quality control of ultrasound use and amniocentesis in individual centres. So it's very difficult for women to find out whether or not the person performing their amniocentesis is adequately trained and competent. Diane Parnell was unlucky. When she went for her amniocentesis, she was scanned before, but not during, the procedure: 'The gynaecologist came in and looked at the scan picture that had been taken minutes before . . . the needle was inserted into my womb and then Terry [her husband] said: "It's failed, he's going to have to do it again." Same problem, same pain if not more, and blood swirling round in the syringe.'

Diane did not miscarry, but her daughter Mishka was born blind and deaf, with severe brain damage. There was a large scar on the scalp, right over where the damage was. Mishka died when she was two. The hospital admitted the amnio was done badly, but they insisted the needle could not have caused Mishka's brain damage. The Parnells turned for help to Oxford pathologist Waney Squier, who has now done a study of brain scans and slides taken from Mishka and other children with similar injuries. She has linked developmental damage precisely to the time of the amniocentesis in each case.

Many obstetricians won't acknowledge the huge variation in

miscarriage rates or the brain damage that can result from botched amniocentesis. At present, the only way of ensuring it isn't done blind is for patients themselves to do quality checks on doctors. This is incredibly difficult. A woman who is already petrified she might have a baby with a congenital abnormality, lies on her back and faces an obstetrician with a needle. Is she going to ask if continuous ultrasound guidance is being used? Recently, I was contacted by two women, one from Manchester whose amniocentesis was done blind by a consultant who didn't speak to her and drew blood on two occasions before giving up. But another woman due to have an amniocentesis at the Alexandra Healthcare NHS Trust in Redditch found out the consultant she was offered did it blind and insisted on seeing someone else.

She eventually got good treatment, but only by asserting herself. Most women are frightened of challenging doctors, as the horrific injuries inflicted by Kent gynaecologist Rodney Ledward will testify. He was dubbed 'the Butcher' by his colleagues at William Harvey Hospital in Ashford. They had to repair his cockups and yet they didn't stop him operating in the first place. Likewise, the majority of competent obstetricians in this country who are doing amniocentesis properly are aware of those in their department who aren't. But will they stop them? No. As ever, the secretive self-regulation of doctors stinks.

Time to Regulate Perfusionists

19 November 1998

Would you want your life support machine operated by an unregulated technician? Probably not. Yet the perfusionists who operate heart-lung bypass machines during open-heart surgery on babies, children and adults have no regulation at all. This fact hit the press recently after a baby undergoing surgery at Guy's Hospital bled to death in seconds when a heart bypass machine modified by an unsupervised trainee perfusionist suffered a catastrophic failure. Four-month-old Hannah Shepherd died after a tube connecting her to the machine 'blew off and whirled around the room,' covering the floor in blood. Hannah was pronounced dead twenty minutes later.

Describing Hannah's death as 'violent and shocking', Dr Selena Lynch, the Southwark coroner, called on the Government to urgently consider imposing registration and regulation controls on the operators of heart-lung bypass machines to minimise the chance of it happening again. She is preparing a report to send to the Department of Health. This plea, however, is old news to the DoH. For some years, perfusionists themselves have applied to become regulated under the Council for the Professions Supplementary to Medicine. A submission in June 1996 was made by the Perfusion Liaison Group of the Society of Perfusionists of Great Britain and Ireland comprising, amongst others Magdi Yacoub, Professor of Cardiac Surgery at the Royal Brompton Hospital and other eminent cardiac surgeons and anaesthetists. It failed. At every stage, obstacles were presented by none other than the Department of Health.

A First-Class Service?

2 December 1998

Frank Dobson's promise to deliver a first-class NHS that is 'modern, dependable and free of all the gross inequalities, variable standards and treatments by postcode that have blighted it for over 50 years' is laudable enough, but how? The *Eye* has exposed alarming variations in the quality of care for all sorts of surgery, but they are equally alarming in general practice. A recent audit of the use of cholesterol-lowering drugs (statins) for GPs in the south-east found a 98-fold variation in prescription.

The key to ensuring a uniform, high-quality service is adequate resources, good training and systematic audit. The latter clearly shows that more complex care needs to be centralised to specialist centres, but no-one takes much notice of audit. Professor Karl Sikora, a cancer specialist at the Hammersmith Hospital, believes 15,000 cancer patients die unnecessarily each year because they aren't treated in specialist cancer centres: 'To get the best possible care, to get the best possible results, to have the best possible chance of surviving you have to make sure that all the expertise is given to you. You can only get that if you see someone that's dealing with a large number of patients with cancer and preferably part of a team that's dealing with specific cancer such as that of the breast or the lung. It's very disheartening for me as a professional to know that we have the skill in this country to treat people very effectively and yet 15,000 people or more are dying each year because they're not getting the best possible cancer care.' Despite the Calman recommendations ordering a reorganisation of cancer care in 1996, the improvements have been blighted by 'insufficient funds, inappropriate management and doctors refusing to change.'

The latest example of audit that has failed to deliver improvements comes from the Royal College of Psychiatrists. They looked at the provision in England and Wales of Electroconvulsive therapy, an effective treatment used for intractable depression when other methods have failed. Despite two previous audits (the last in 1991) and clear Royal College standards, only a third of clinics met them in 1996, when the audit finished. Only 16% of consultants were able to attend ECT sessions and supervise their juniors, 41% had out dated machines and two thirds had no clear policies to help guide junior doctors to administer ECT effectively.

In Scotland, however, the junior staff receive excellent training, the consultants are present at ECT sessions, EEG (brain wave) monitoring with modern equipment is freely available and an audit of outcomes has revealed that over 70% of patients improve after ECT. How can Scotland succeed where England and Wales are failing? Is it resources (Scotland gets more funding per head than the population down south), is it working conditions, or are Scottish psychiatrists a more conscientious and patient-serving bunch?

Another Scottish audit of infertility treatment is less favourable. 80% of men with low sperm counts being treated by consultant urologists are given anti-oestrogen drugs, despite good proof from a 1986 World Health Organisation trial that they are of no benefit. Indeed, low sperm count is still notoriously difficult to treat and yet couples are languishing in urology clinics with time ticking away, when their best chance of success lies in a prompt referral for assisted conception.

So, what is Mr Dobson to do with doctors who ignore audit, guidelines and evidence? Hit them with a stick or give them the resources to do it? At present, his mind may be elsewhere. When I met him at an NHS 50th-anniversary celebration, he was trying to pin down a surgeon in middle-England who goes by the name of 'The Terminator'. That, alas, is insufficient to stop him. Why? He doesn't audit his work, so it's very hard to gather the evidence.

Poor Stroke Services

28 December 1998

What's the single main cause of disability in the UK? What's the third biggest killer? And what's being done about it? Stroke, stroke and not much. Each year 100,000 people suffer a stroke – that's one every five minutes – with often devastating consequences. 5.8% of the entire NHS and social services budget is spent on treatment, and most of that goes on 'rehabilitation'. Fortunately, there is good evidence that patients treated in specialist units do better. Back in 1993, the *Lancet*[1] published an overview of all the randomised controlled trials between 1962 and 1993 comparing specialist stroke management with non-specialist. Patients treated in stroke units were 28% more likely to be alive after four months and 21% more likely to make it to a year. In nine out of ten of the units, the patients also achieved 'functional gains' (i.e. were less disabled after treatment).

In 1997, the *British Medical Journal* published a similar review which found that specialist stroke care reduced the chances of dying or remaining physically dependent by 29%.[2] If all patients had access to such care, over 4,500 lives a year would be saved and another 6,250 patients would regain independence, compared to conventional care. There is no increase in the use of resources with such care and there is some evidence that hospital stays may be shorter. There is also the potential for huge savings in that many thousands of patients would not need long-term institutional care nor draw disability benefits, and the burden on carers, who currently put in 3.7 million hours a week, would be much reduced.

The Department of Health has at least recognised that stroke care is a problem, costing £2.3 billion a year with patients occupying 20% of acute hospital beds and 25% of long-term beds. The Government's 'Our Healthier Nation' targets include a reduction in the death rate from heart disease and stroke amongst those under 65 by a further third. However, despite a recent report by the Clinical Standards Advisory Group that found widespread variations in stroke treatment

[1] *Lancet* 1993; 342: 395–8.
[2] *BMJ* 1997; 314: 1151–9.

and care, the Government has yet to announce any national implementation for organised stroke care. If such a scheme had been implemented in 1993 when the evidence of benefit was clear, many thousands of stroke patients would have been alive and free from disability.

At present, the stroke care you or your relatives receive is a postcode lottery, with those who make it to a specialist unit 29% more likely to survive and regain independence. If there is no such unit in your area, you (or your relatives) should insist on being taken to one.

A League of Their Own

The Government's much-trumpeted NHS league tables have turned out to be very incomplete. More than half the 'clinical indicators' promised in July 1997 have failed to make an appearance. Measures of hospital acquired infections, a range of surgical complications and deaths in hospital after surgery are conspicuous by their absence. In truth, most of us still working in the 'modern, dependable' NHS still bumble on without much idea of how we're doing. Happy New Year.

Private Malpractice

30 January 1999

At present, anyone can call themselves a consultant in cosmetic surgery, open a clinic and perform surgery, provided they don't claim to have a medical degree. And a physiotherapist struck off by his or her regulatory body (the Register of the Council for the Professions Supplementary to Medicine) can open a private clinic that afternoon and practise as a . . . er . . . physiotherapist. And even though doctors in private practice are within the remit of GMC regulation, very few are called to account for misconduct. Anyone, however slim, can obtain amphetamines for weight loss from doctors in private slimming clinics. And wealthy addicts worried about their next fix can pop off to Harley Street and buy whatever they want. The doctor gains a huge fee for the consultation and the pharmacist gets a huge mark-up on the prescription. All grossly unethical but entirely legal.

Even 'routine' private practice is open to widespread abuse. Because of the pecuniary incentive to investigate or operate, patients may be given unnecessary tests or treatments or, just as alarming, be operated on by surgeons with no expertise in that particular area. In a letter to the *BMJ* (Vol. 317, p. 811 [September 19, 1998]), obstetrician Beverley Webb, chairman of the medical advisory committee at Pinehill Hospital, Hitchin, Hertfordshire wrote:

'Unnecessary operations are a great problem, some being performed by doctors who have had only basic training in the techniques while they were passing though a specialty. . . . What does one do if a colleague who is not an orthopaedic surgeon or hand surgeon operates on Dupytren's contractures, or a colleague who is not a plastic surgeon performs breast reductions, or a colleague who is not a gynaecologist inappropriately operates on genital prolapse? What do you do if a colleague always finds something to operate on no matter what the patient is referred with? And what do you say to the anaesthetist who always puts in a regional block as well as giving a general anaesthetic in order to bump up the fee?

'It astounds me that the medical insurance companies themselves have not policed these sorts of activities in order to reduce their own financial outgoings. All of these examples are observed every week by all of us who have our eyes open. Worse, they are obvious to our nursing and paramedical colleagues, who wonder why we are doing nothing to correct these anomalies . . .' Alas, if a cockup occurs in private practice (and this is increasingly common according to a report by Action for Victims of Medical Accidents), patients don't have recourse to the NHS complaints or compensation procedures.

Stroke and More

12 February 1999

Recently, the *Eye* reported that access to specialist stroke units for each of the 100,000 patients who suffer a stroke each year would save over 4,500 lives a year and drastically reduce the disability suffered by survivors. Continuing the theme, Labour MP Harry Barnes asked health secretary Frank Dobson: 'what right stroke victims or their relatives have to insist on patients' treatment in specialist stroke units?' The written answer from health minister John Hutton (*Hansard*, January 25, 1999) was illuminating: 'Following a stroke, patients are entitled to expect that an appropriate service will be provided but that service will not necessarily be within a specialist stroke unit. The organisation of health authorities services, including those of people who have had a stroke, and the manner in which they are delivered are matters for the health authority taking account of the needs of the local population and the priorities set for the use of the available resources.'

A classic piece of buck passing and, given that patients in specialist stroke units do much better than those who aren't, a direct contradiction of the Government White Paper *A First Class Service: Quality in the New NHS* published last year. Here Mr Dobson enthuses that 'all patients should receive a first class service. The unacceptable variations that have grown up in recent years must end.' Given that stroke is the commonest cause of disability in the UK and the third biggest killer, it would seem a reasonable place to start. Alas, Mr Dobson seems pretty clueless as to the current state of stroke care. Mr Barnes asked him for his estimate of the money spent on stroke care each year, the percentage of the NHS budget used, how many specialist stroke units there are, how many patients are treated in them and an estimate of their effectiveness. The answer? 'The information requested is not available.'

Given the patchy quality of care in the NHS, doctors are resorting to putting in writing what they'd insist on if they got ill. In the *Lancet* (Vol. 352, October 1998), Dr Kennedy R Lees from Glasgow's Western Infirmary gives us a paper entitled 'If I had a stroke . . .'. Says Dr Lees 'I would choose a hospital with an expressed interest in stroke and preferably an acute-stroke unit.' And so should everyone (although it's hard to choose when you've had a massive stroke).

More controversy from the *Lancet*, where Dr John G F Cleland from the Department of Cardiology at Hull's Castle Hill Hospital has described the death of patients with heart failure who didn't have access to 'inexpensive and cost-effective treatment' as 'involuntary euthanasia' (Vol. 352, 29 August, 1998). Strong words, but the evidence that putting such patients on drugs called ACE inhibitors reduces their chance of death is equally strong. We've known this for many years and yet a lot of patients are still denied treatment. In America, this would be cause for legal action; in the UK we accept whatever the NHS gives us.

However, the involuntary euthanasia tag is a dangerous one, given that it would apply to every area of medicine, where some patients are denied life-saving treatment which is readily available to others (e.g. acute stroke care). If everyone who's had a heart attack, angina, stroke or mini-stroke took an aspirin every day they'd reduce their risk of death. Alas, at present, only half of them do and so an estimated 13,400 people each year are dying unnecessarily. Is this involuntary euthanasia?

If every patient with high blood pressure received effective treatment, if every smoker had access to advice and nicotine-replacement therapy, if those with heart disease and high cholesterol were given statins (cholesterol-lowering drugs), if all those over 65 had a flu jab . . . Each year, many thousands of lives could be saved. Not only that, but in each case treatment is likely to save money when compared to the cost of treatment after the disease strikes (although unnecessary death is, ultimately, very cheap if you can hide it from a lawyer).

The Royal College of Surgeons Awakes

25 February 1999
The Children's Liver Disease Foundation and national media have supported the *Eye*'s call for the Kasai operation to be limited to specialist centres. This has forced a U-turn from the Royal College of Surgeons, which has now added its support and put considerable pressure on the Department of Health.

The Kasai operation can fail even at the best centres but, if it does, they have the expert support team of hepatologists, pathologists, anaesthetists, nurses and nutritionists who can then get the baby as fit as possible for liver transplant. At some non-specialist centres, the failed Kasai operations aren't being picked up quickly and the babies die before they have liver transplants.

Professor Ted Howard, the UK's leading Kasai surgeon, stresses the importance of training: 'It is a very complicated operation and to do it well, you need to be operating in and around the liver all the time. You simply can't expect general paediatric surgeons who operate in the liver once a year to get good results. The same applies to surgery for liver cancer – I'm sure the same huge variation in care is occurring.'

The current situation is indefensible and makes no financial sense either. The Kasai operation, done well or badly, costs around £8,000 but, if it fails, a liver transplant will cost up to £75,000. Given the national shortage of donor livers, some babies may die before a suitable transplant can be found, and others will use a liver that could have been given to another patient if the operation had been done properly in the first place. And transplantation itself is not without risks.

Even at the best centres, 10–20% of babies die within three years and those that survive have to take life-long immuno-suppressive drugs and risk long-term complication of liver rejection. There are only 50 babies a year born with biliary atresia and there is simply no excuse for not centralising the service to three or four specialist centres. In a press release, the Department of Health admitted that it had known about the scandal for fourteen years. Now, with a nudge from the *Eye*, it may finally be forced to act.

Why Babies Still Die

10 March 1999
In 1997, the *British Medical Journal* (Vol. 315, July 19, 1997) reported that half of the deaths of young infants each year might be avoidable. 1,266 infant deaths were investigated and the report concluded that in 52% of cases, different care 'would reasonably have been expected to have made a difference' and in a further 25% of cases it 'might have made a difference'.

Doctors delivered suboptimal care in 60% of cases, with hospital midwives implicated in 46%. Only 20% of cases involved consultants or senior midwives, and the report recommended improved supervision of junior staff to reduce deaths. It also called for nationally approved assessment and accreditation of the relevant staff.

A year later, the fifth annual *Confidential Enquiry into Stillbirths and Deaths* confirmed that some babies die due to 'poor clinical management'. Many of the babies who died had been ill enough to warrant medical attention in the 24 hours before they died, but appropriate action wasn't taken. As ever, you get the NHS you pay for. If the Government believes its own hype of a first-class NHS, it needs to fund enough consultant posts for doctors-in-training to have round-the-clock supervision. If it prefers to muddle along with patchy care and hundreds of preventable child deaths each year, then Dobson should at least make this explicit.

Unnecessary Intervention?

7 April 1998

Sandra Simkin, from the Campaign Against Hysterectomy and Unnecessary Operations on Women (CAHUOW), is not convinced that we need more consultant obstetricians: 'It is interesting that you cite perinatal and neonatal deaths as a reason to create more consultant jobs and provide work for these doctors. The statutory responsibility for maternity care lies with midwives, not obstetricians, and the crisis surrounding maternity services is not about the supply of obstetricians, but the lack of midwives.

'Ever since the management of maternity services was grabbed by obstetricians there has been a measurable falling off in the service to mothers and a massive increase in obstetric intervention including drugs, episiotomies and caesarean sections. ... The over-supply of obstetricians has allowed thousands of unnecessary hysterectomies to co-exist with a caesarean-section rate which is more than a third in excess of the World Health Organisation standard. ... If unnecessary surgery on women was stopped now, all pretension of a staffing crisis would also cease.'

Mrs Simkin acknowledges that there is a need for an

emergency obstetric service, and indeed most of the studies of preventable death in and around childbirth call for both more senior midwives and obstetricians to supervise junior staff. However, even obstetricians admit that high-tech medical involvement can result in over-use of the scalpel. Continuous electronic (CTG) monitoring of uterine contractions and the baby's heart rate is routinely used for low-risk deliveries and yet trials have repeatedly found little benefit for these women and an increased risk of surgery. As consultant Donald Gibb from London's King's Hospital puts it: 'Electronic monitoring has certainly led to an increase in caesarean sections. This may have been due to failure of the technique during its introduction but in every hospital where you start doing it, you immediately put up the caesarean section rate.'

In the past 30 years, the caesarean section rate in the UK has risen from 5% to 17% and in some areas it is much higher (e.g. 28% in Bromsgrove). One study found that 31% of London's female obstetricians would routinely opt for the operation for themselves, mainly because they wished to avoid damage to the vagina, anus and pelvic floor muscles. But a planned caesarean section is three times as life-threatening to the mother as a normal birth (although the risks are still low), and complications include adhesions, intestinal obstruction, bladder injury and possible uterine rupture next time around. These risks obviously vary with the experience and skill of the surgical team.

Some hospitals have labour wards staffed entirely by midwives (e.g. the Liverpool Women's Hospital) and the 'intervention rate' in such units is lower and resources are saved (caesareans cost, on average, £760). However, smaller maternity units are having to fight for survival and when the unit at Ashford in Middlesex closed in 1996, the local caesarean rate rose. In 1995, a survey by the National Childbirth Trust found that 99% of women surveyed said their local small unit provided nicer, more personalised care for low-risk women.

And their record on supporting breast-feeding is particularly strong. As for very low-tech home-births, which constitute less than 2% of all deliveries, a study by the NHS Centre for Reviews and Dissemination concluded: 'There is no evidence that hospital births are safer for all women and all babies, as long as there are no serious complications during pregnancy.'

Mrs Simkin's final charge – that more gynaecologists means more hysterectomies – also has a ring of truth, but the problem of heavy periods (menorrhagia) starts with inadequate medical treatment. Many women are still given norethisterone, a drug which is no better in the long term than a placebo. When it doesn't work, they get referred for surgery which they may have avoided if they'd had an effective drug first (e.g. tranexamic or mefenamic acid). As for the surgery itself, you're fifteen times more likely to have a hysterectomy if you've got no secondary education. As a (male) gynaecologist wrote in the *British Medical Journal*: 'removing the wombs of low-income women is often more efficient than taking the time to educate them and treat them medically.' There is, however, one group of middle-class patients where hysterectomies are also common. The wives of gynaecologists.

A Victory for the *Eye*

6 May 1999

Last August, the *Eye* suggested that babies with biliary atresia should be treated at either Birmingham, Leeds or King's, London – the three expert centres treating enough patients to produce statistically meaningful results. Nine months later, Frank Dobson agrees. In a press release from the Department of Health (April 30), the health secretary has agreed with all of the *Eye*'s proposals.

Not everyone is happy. In a letter to the *British Medical*

Journal, five consultants from Booth Hall Children's Hospital and Royal Manchester Children's Hospital have complained that the *Eye*'s coverage was 'inaccurate and misleading' (*BMJ*, April 10). Manchester was a 'medium-volume centre' with an average success rate of 54% and, if biliary atresia was a common disease, it might well have been chosen as another specialist centre. However, with only 50 cases a year there is only a need for three such centres. Any more would dilute the expertise and make any audit much less reliable.

The argument that parents want their babies to be treated locally rather than travel further was dismissed by the Children's Liver Disease Foundation. As chief executive Catherine Arkley put it: 'Parents would move to hell and back to get the best for their children.' I have also spoken to the parents of children who had unsuccessful surgery at local non-specialist centres without knowing that such a disparity in results existed. They feel outrage and guilt that this information was not made available to them (when it has been apparent since 1984).

The Manchester team were clearly providing a much better service than those doing just one operation a year and are angry that the debate has been held in the media rather than behind the closed doors of the profession. Consultants at Birmingham Children's Hospital are also annoyed that their audit was published first in the *Eye* rather than the *Lancet*. Professional journals like to have first bite, and if something has been leaked to the media first, they will often refuse to publish.

However, the information came from concerned doctors working in the field who felt the public-interest element was so strong, it was worth risking a breach of confidentiality and professional censure to get it into the public domain. The latest biliary atresia audit had been sitting on desks since 1996 and, aside from minor statistical adjustments, is as the *Eye* published it. The profession may have eventually got round to weeding out the surgeons who were attempting rare, complex operations on babies and getting demonstrably poor results, but the public exposure of this scandal – admittedly painful for some parents – has had a huge impact on speeding up the process.

As ever, the whistleblowers must insist on remaining anonymous for fear of reprisals. Little has changed in the seven years since Bristol, except perhaps that the Royal College of Surgeons moves a little quicker. It was the first professional body to act on the biliary atresia audit. However, its president, Barry Jackson, refutes the *Eye*'s claim that the Royal College of Surgeons knows the identity of poorly performing surgeons through its confidential audits. The claim was based on a 1996 interview given by an RCS spokesman, the late Brendan Devlin, who told BBC2's *Trust Me I'm A Doctor* that he was aware of the identity of 'No. 169', a surgeon with very poor results for prostate surgery.

'I can state now – unequivocally – that the college has never known the identity of No. 169,' writes Mr Jackson. 'Brendan Devlin did, as the then director of the Comparative Audit Service, but this was privileged information.' Alas, he's now dead. As for the *Eye*'s other question (what's the point of spending millions on audit if you can't identify the poor performers and prove to the public they've been sorted out?), Mr Jackson has promised to reply shortly in greater detail. In the meantime, No. 169 could still be out there. Look for a tattoo behind the left ear.

Brain Surgery Special

4 June 1999
'Blair plan aims to cut cancer deaths by a fifth', declared *The Times* on May 21 (p. 8). This headline was ironically juxtaposed with the separate story of 'Tumour girl's life-saving flight'. The parents of Holly Crisp, aged eight, raised £40,000 for their

daughter to be treated by Patrick Kelly at the New York University Medical Centre because they were unable to find an equivalent standard of neurosurgery in the UK. This raises two important questions. Is the standard of UK neurosurgery for childhood brain tumours significantly worse than in America? And if so, do parents and patients have a right to an extra-contractual referral to a centre of proven excellence, funded by the NHS, if they are unable to find an acceptable standard of treatment in their own district or country?

In the UK, the campaign to make parents of children with brain tumours aware of the wide variations in treatment success from different centres has been spearheaded by Faye McCluckie. Mrs McCluckie's daughter was deemed to have an inoperable tumour by UK surgeons in 1994. Her consultant at the time agreed that he lacked the expertise to do the operation, but recommended treatment by Professor Kelly in New York. As a result of this recommendation, the NHS funded the cost of the treatment.

Professor Kelly's expertise stems from a number of factors. Not only does he have the latest computer-assisted image-guided equipment to aid minimally invasive surgery but – crucially – he has the expertise and experience to use it, operating on some 350 patients a year. In the UK, not only is the equipment sometimes absent or obsolete but the service has yet to be centralised into a few expert centres. Hence, some surgeons are doing too few of the operations to gain the expertise or produce statistically meaningful results.

As for the long-term survival prospects of the children, a recent study conducted by the Pediatric Brain Tumor Program in America found that 'if the surgeon leaves more than about ¼ teaspoon of detectable tumour, the survival rate drops from 78% to approximately 53%.' The best chance of survival is clearly to go to a centre that treats lots of children and openly publishes its results. Alas, your chance of an extra-contractual referral if such a service is not available locally depends not on your surgeon's published record of competence, which may not exist, but on his opinion of whether he is capable of attempting the surgery. These are clearly not the same thing.

As with all life-threatening treatment, you should ask to see an audit of the results and how they compare nationally and, possibly, internationally. If such information is not forthcoming or otherwise unsatisfactory, you have a strong case with your health authority for an extra-contractual referral to a centre that can prove its competence.

Heart Surgery Today

18 June 1999

There are currently 35 units performing cardiac surgery in the UK and just one of them publishes its results for both adult and child surgery on the internet – Bristol (see www.ubht.org.uk). The child surgery results are mercifully excellent, thanks to the appointment of surgeon Ash Pawade, several specialist intensivists and the reorganisation of the service onto a single site.

However, the spirit of openness now evident in Bristol is by no means universal. For 1997–98, 10 of the 35 units didn't even submit audit figures to the database at all. In some cases, the trust itself is reluctant to make the investment in the software and personnel training needed to collect the data, but the Bristol team has proved that these costs are relatively small in terms of time and money and hence this is inexcusable. It may also be that cardiac surgery is still peppered with dinosaurs who don't feel they should open up their performance to outside scrutiny.

Those hospitals who were unable to contribute to the audit include Plymouth's Derriford Hospital, Sheffield's Northern

General, Southampton General, North Staffordshire Royal Infirmary in Stoke-on-Trent, London's Royal Hospitals Trust, Oxford Heart Centre, Aberdeen Royal Infirmary, Belfast's Royal Victoria Infirmary and both the Royal Infirmary and Western Infirmary in Glasgow.

What, No Midwife?

26 August 1999

In 1993, the Conservative Government launched *Changing Childbirth*, a project aimed at increasing the choices given to pregnant women about their maternity care. Six years later, an audit of 87% of the midwifery units in England has found that only three can deliver the quality of care promised in the report. The vast majority of units were short of midwives, with as many as eighteen vacant posts in some London trusts and 30% of units unable to provide 'one-to-one' care for women in labour. The national shortfall of midwives needed to get all units up to standard is estimated at 5,000 but amidst the Government's £5 million nurse-recruitment campaign, the only ads for midwifery were on local radio. Unsurprisingly, the Department of Health has no idea how many midwives it has attracted back to work.

The DoH does, however, have a better idea of how many it's losing. Two thousand have gone in the last three years, leaving the current level at its lowest for ten years. The latest high-profile loss is Fiona Sommerville, head of midwifery services at Brighton Health Care NHS Trust, who is going because 'cuts have caused a growing conflict between my professional role and my managerial role. . . . I have struggled to maintain the quality of service at a level I feel patients deserve . . . the trust has no more money. In fact, it needs to make a saving of £1.5

million this year. Midwifery is not a priority because it does not attract waiting list money.'

Last month, the National Childbirth Trust expressed its 'bitter disappointment' that many women are still being denied home births despite evidence that for low-risk pregnancies you're just as safe (if not safer) at home. In fact, the decision about where to have a baby rests entirely with the mother, but if you do it without a good midwife, you're really tempting fate. Alas, many home-birthers buy the plastic sheeting and the cord cutter only to be told their midwife has been cancelled at the last minute due to staff shortages. They then rush into hospital to be offered half a trainee midwife and a medical student. So much for changing childbirth.

ALAN MILBURN
October 1999–June 2003

Alan Milburn, affectionately known as 'Bastard', was in the ideal situation to break a few windows. He had a clutch of medical scandals (Bristol, Shipman, Alder Hey, assorted rogue gynaecologists) to use as evidence to tighten control over doctors, and enough money to sweeten the pill of a market reform programme that was beyond Thatcher's dreams. He was the Marmite health minister – loathed or loved.

Milburn's baptism was one of the worst winters on record, but the bad press included Lord Winston's tirade about his mother's treatment which bounced Blair into announcing that NHS funding would match the European average. He pushed through Labour's NHS Plan on the pretence that it was built around the needs of patients, rather than a veiled invitation to let private competition into the NHS. Doctors didn't spot the deception until too late, because we didn't understand management jargon like 'additionality', 'contestability' and 'introducing diversity into provision'.

Milburn's undoing was his attempt to micromanage the NHS from the centre with impatient haste. He threw so much shit at the walls that some of it had to stick, but as none of his reforms was piloted or evaluated, it's hard to say which bits. Lots of tough targets were set, and lots of figures were fiddled to meet them. Thanks to the Bristol Inquiry report, Milburn introduced standards, inspections and some measure of quality control into the NHS, but it was aggressively, centrally imposed. Many doctors saw him as a bully and he struggled to get them onside, which could be one reason why he suddenly gave up to spend more time at home. The lesson? You can't run the NHS or a family from Whitehall. And doctors want time for their children too.

PRIVATE EYE
Accepting the Buck

21 October 1999

Frank Dobson's swift and unseemly departure from the Department of Health was not only, it seems, to spike Ken Livingstone's mayoral ambitions. Prime Minister Blair's dream of unleashing a radical health agenda on the 'dark forces of Conservatism' (i.e. the BMA) would not have sat well with Dobson's Old Labour beliefs. So enter Alan 'Modernisation is here to stay' Milburn, whose recent stint as health minister led to him being branded 'anti-doctor' by Professor John Ward, vice-president of the Royal College of Physicians. The BMA's Dr Peter Hawker invited him to 'stop attacking the profession and defend doctors' performance'. Mr Milburn took no notice at all and, now he's in charge, he'll take on the medical profession in ways that Margaret Thatcher wouldn't have dared. But is he prepared to take ultimate responsibility for the quality of care in the NHS?

The *Eye*'s repeated exposure of surgical scandals has shown how reluctant the Department of Health has been to accept responsibility without the agreement of the Royal Colleges, which are deeply self-protective and self-serving. If Milburn tries to wrestle control away from the medical profession, he can be sure his civil servants will not be lining up behind him to accept it. And the General Medical Council only launches itself into action years after the event, to save its skin. The GMC gets away with it because no-one else wants to take on responsibility for regulating doctors, especially when most of our cockups are tied up with lack of manpower, training and resources. As Mr Milburn will soon find out, you get the health service you pay for and the doctors you deserve.

A good start would be to collect, learn from and publish outcomes so at least we know what we're dealing with. Recently, the Audit Commission published *Critical to Success*, a report into the quality of care in intensive care units in England and Wales. Death rates vary greatly, with some units having thrice the average mortality. Do we know the good ones? Do we know the bad ones? Do we have any guarantee that the bad ones will be sorted out? Do we buggery. It had to be kept a secret 'to encourage units to participate'. So much for freedom of information.

Who Picks Up Doctors' Mistakes?

18 November 1999

Can you make the NHS safer from the top down? We now have a National Institute for Clinical Excellence (NICE) to sift through the evidence and decide on what the NHS should (and shouldn't) provide, and the Commission for Health Improvement, to ensure that NICE's diktats are observed. The commission's first job has been to change its acronym from CHIMP (the ape-association was deemed too flippant) to CHI (half a celebrity panda).

Whether either of these quangos will change behaviour on the ground is debatable. For over ten years Dr William Pickering, a GP with wide experience of medico-legal work, has campaigned for an independent medical inspectorate by asking 'who picks up doctors' mistakes?' Pickering has concentrated on the very basic and rudimentary clinical errors that any reasonably competent doctor should avoid. These generally involve the unnecessarily late diagnosis of treatable disease and the improper supervision of ongoing medical treatment.

In his medico-legal work, Pickering has seen repeated examples of doctors of all ages and ranks failing to follow basic medical rules. For example, failing to investigate blood in the urine resulting in death from undiagnosed bladder cancer or failure to put a patient with a heart attack or a stroke on medication to prevent a further attack. Errors such as these happen every day in the NHS but even when they result in patient harm, they are rarely picked up or commented on. Even at the simplest of levels, there is no systematic way of identifying and acting on doctors' individual mistakes.

Pickering believes that an independent medical inspectorate, headed by doctors with a presence in every region, would be a huge step forward. Only doctors have the easy access to patient records necessary to make an informed judgement, and they have a much clearer idea of what is acceptable practice. The inspectors would not, however, be employed by the NHS and would therefore be less likely to let misguided loyalty get in the way of rational thought. Just an idea.

Gagging for a Lord

10 January 2000
This year's NHS winter crisis had the added spice of Lord Winston's diatribe in the *New Statesman* about how we spend even less of our GDP on health than Poland. This after his mother fell, unobserved, out of an NHS bed. Tony Blair's response has been to bully the good Lord into a retraction, perhaps with the threat of a complaint to the GMC (for divulging that heavily pregnant Cherie has decided not to push and pant). But Winston at least panicked Blair into promising to raise NHS funding to European levels.

Winston need not have retracted. Any genuine concern he raises about the NHS should be protected by the Public Interest Disclosure Act, which became law last July to prevent the persecution of whistleblowers. And everyone knows Cherie Blair had a caesarean section last time round and so is highly likely to have another given her age. They might even shave a little of her pubic hair off prior to the incision. This amounts to nothing more than informed speculation and – given that Winston is not in any way involved in her medical care – this does not constitute a breach of confidentiality.

Alas, politicians suffused with self-importance seem incapable of making this distinction. In July 1998, Gregor Mackay – then press secretary to William Hague – reported me directly to the GMC for disrespectful speculation about the Leader of the Opposition's prolonged absence from work: 'I thought the article highly unprofessional and a poor advert for your profession,' fumed Mackay, who was sacked shortly afterwards. After due consideration, the GMC concluded that as I have never been Mr Hague's doctor, my comments were of no interest to them. Ditto Lord Winston and Cherie. Even if she's having it on all fours in Lord Archer's Jacuzzi.

Fortunately, nurses seem less inclined than Lord Winston to be gagged. As community nurse Barbara Mathews from Swansea writes in the *Nursing Times*, 'I am frequently appalled by the basic lack of nursing care for some of my older patients in hospital. They develop painful pressure sores that take months to heal. Drinks are placed out of reach, false teeth not cleaned, food left untouched. I know staff levels are low, but they always were.'

And that's the point. This winter has been no different to every winter in the NHS, in terms of the level of sickness. However, many NHS staff swallowed Labour's trite 'things can only get better' line and believed that, a few years into office, they genuinely would. The fact that so little has changed in the NHS has led to widespread disillusionment, with a knock-on effect on patient care. Lord Winston is just the tip of a very angry iceberg.

Trust Me, I'm Still A Doctor

3 February 2000

Harold Shipman is free to doctor his fellow prisoners, despite his fifteen murder convictions, since the GMC is prohibited from taking action while a criminal investigation proceeds, and will be further delayed if Shipman appeals. Once criminal proceedings are completed, the GMC is then required to give 28 days' notice of the intention to suspend a doctor from the register. So Shipman can call himself a doctor for some while yet.

Many doctors now have little faith in the GMC's ability to regulate the profession. As Dr Bill Pickering writes: 'One important reason that Shipman got away with it for so long was because he knew that in the NHS, and in general practice in particular, doctors can do more or less what they like. They call it "clinical freedom" and cherish it. No one (except the law) can meaningfully challenge their actions, and then only if they are found out. Medical ethics do not include commenting on another doctor's practice, nor do they insist upon an open mentality. The "self-regulation" of doctors is, therefore, equivalent to no regulation.'

Unaffordable Drugs

17 February 2000

Last July, the board of the Royal Surrey Hospital NHS Trust asked their solicitors for advice on behalf of consultants who were unable to prescribe expensive drugs for the treatment of ovarian cancer because their budget for such treatments had been cut by £150,000. The consultants wanted to know whether they should tell patients the truth: 'There is a drug that might help you but we can't afford it.' Or whether to resort to kind but dishonest paternalism: 'There is no effective treatment for you.'

The Trust could have afforded the drug eighteen months previously, but is now £1.4 million in the red. As Professor Hilary Thomas, a cancer specialist, put it: 'I have patients who are young and relatively fit and I have a dilemma about whether I am completely honest with them and leave them with the awful thought that if they were private patients, they would be offered the drug.' The Trust's solicitors advised that doctors should always be entirely open and honest with patients, even if it leaves Prof. Thomas with some tough consultations. One patient of his was denied the drug (Hycamtin or topotecan) and died shortly afterwards. He then had to face her husband knowing she hadn't been given the best possible chance of living.

Elsewhere, the information given to patients about ovarian cancer drugs still varies widely between consultants. As a Bristol cancer specialist told me last week: 'One consultant won't mention the ovarian cancer drugs at all if there is no funding for them, because it's cruel. In effect, you're saying, "There is a drug that may help you and it is available in some parts of the NHS but not this one, so tough." The second consultant tells patients these drugs exist to allow the rich ones to buy them privately and the poor ones to go to the papers and try to raise the money in a campaign (which is usually too late to be successful). And the third consultant tells patients that they can't have the drugs and they should lobby their MPs.'

If patients have a right to information about effective treatments their health authority won't pay for, do they also have a right to know about centres of excellence their health authority won't send them to? A recurring problem the *Eye* has repeatedly exposed is that non-specialist units which lack the expertise and resources to do complex procedures continue to do so, and are effectively protected from accountability because the numbers of patients they treat are so small as to be statistically meaningless. But what if a surgeon was obliged to say: 'I only do a couple of these a year, my results mean nothing but I'd like to have a go anyway. And by the way, there's a specialist centre a hundred miles away where they do lots of these, have all the resources and specialist staff and get statistically good results. But you can't go there.'

A few operations are designated to specialist centres, which should guarantee funding, and the Government also has a scheme to allow health authorities to fund treatments outside their area with the catchy title of OATS (out-of-area treatment scheme). However, this is, according to a DoH release, intended primarily for emergencies and like everything else in the NHS is severely cash-limited. This rationing, according to Oxford neurosurgeon Tipu Azis, is sowing the seeds for another Bristol: 'For more complex operations, local units are unlikely to ever develop the critical mass of competence that specialist centres have. As in Bristol, there is a very real risk that a relatively inexperienced team could produce unacceptable results.

'Some procedures are done locally two or three times a year, when I do them two or three times a week. The Government is hypocritical in that it criticised the Bristol heart surgeons yet it is encouraging the same situation to occur in multiple specialties across the country.' Mr Azis, a Labour supporter, has every reason to be angry. In the last few years, referrals to his unit for the treatment of the tremors of Parkinson's disease have plummeted, even though he openly audits his work and has an 80% success rate. His fear is that either patients are not getting the treatment they need – or they may be getting it done badly. Either way, it would be much cheaper to the NHS in the long term to pay for treatment to be done properly in specialist centres first time round.

Penis Dabbling

6 April 2000

In the NHS you can't always have the very best but you at least deserve to avoid the bodgers. Especially when someone's cutting open your penis. Hypospadius is a common condition, affecting around 1% of boys in the UK, and occurs when the urethra doesn't make it to the end of the penis, but opens on the underside. In the right hands, a two-stage operation will restore a perfect functioning penis. In the wrong hands, you end up with something that looks like the butcher's dog has eaten it and sprays urine all over the place. You have to sit down to pee but, being embarrassed and not knowing any alternative options, you grow up accepting this and never have sex.

Aivar Bracka, a plastic surgeon in Stourbridge, specialises in genital reconstruction operations, gets excellent results and has the audit (and photographs) to prove it. His hypospadius operations are a work of art, but about a third of them are 'salvage procedures' – trying to put right the damage done by previous surgery. He showed me a shocking photo of a man who'd had 50 failed operations on his penis. Why did he keep going back? He was ashamed and embarrassed, he wasn't offered another opinion and the hospital staff kept telling him his surgeon was 'a lovely man' and he was in 'good hands'.

In the present system, there's nothing to stop any urologist, paediatric surgeon or general surgeon having a go at once-a-year hypospadius surgery. But as patients or parents very rarely shout the results from the rooftops, the damage is usually kept under wraps. At the age of four, identical twins Henry and Charlie Phipps had failed surgery at a non-specialist centre. They were both in extreme pain after the operation, and Charlie had to be rushed back to theatre to be catheterised – only they didn't have the right-sized catheter so they used a feeding tube. And when he finally came to 'try out his new willy', the urine came out of five holes like a colander. Henry had a similar result.

Sue and Peter Phipps decided to decline the offer of more surgery and went in search of a specialist, ending up with Bracka, who performed a miraculous transformation. But Jake Marshall went under the knife four times before he got to see a specialist. As his mother Sarah put it: 'I just can't describe the feeling that your son's been butchered by somebody. And he shouldn't be allowed to do it.' Fair point.

What No Drugs (Again)?

8 June 2000

In February, the *Eye* reported the dilemma facing cancer specialists in Bristol about whether to tell patients about new drugs that might help them, but can't be afforded on the NHS budget. Some don't mention them, some mention them in the hope that the patient can raise the money to pay for them privately and some advise patients to write to their MP, as if that'll make you live longer. On April 11, Professor Gordon McVie, Director General of the Cancer Research Campaign, decided to give Avon Health Authority a good kicking on the *Today* programme, describing it as 'disgraceful' and 'guilty of hiding behind the lack of evidence'.

McVie is wide of the mark here. If Avon Health Authority is guilty of anything it is honesty, having admitted to the media that it just doesn't have the money to allow specialists to prescribe expensive drugs such as Docetaxel for advanced breast cancer. Most other health authorities hide behind the excuse that 'it's up to individual doctors to decide what drugs they use,' knowing full well they can't use the drugs they want to. The situation is not helped by press reports, repeated on the

BBC website, that Docetaxel is freely available in Somerset. In fact, the residents of both Somerset and Avon can only get the drug on the NHS if they agree to take part in a clinical trial, which could mean they end up with a placebo.

Avon's openness about rationing at least means patients should be deprived of new drugs in a fair way. The ovarian cancer drug Paclitaxel has been used in Avon since 1998 but, as public health consultant Dr Angela Raffle puts it, 'It would be misleading to say Avon has found sufficient new money to fully meet the costs of this.' In the last three years, the funding to the Bristol Oncology Centre has increased by £1.65 million but 'this is not sufficient to keep up with the increase in numbers of patients and the costs of new chemotherapy agents.' McVie can rant about Avon on Radio 4, but perhaps the debate would be better served if he popped down to Bristol and told them in person where to magic the money from.

Meanwhile, at Ealing, Hammersmith and Fulham Mental Health NHS Trust, patients with dementia have been denied two new drugs (Aricept and Reminyl) for Alzheimer's disease. As a consultant who wishes to remain anonymous put it: 'They don't cure Alzheimer's but they do relieve symptoms in many cases and keep people out of institutional care and in the care of their families for longer. Until March, the health authority decided not to increase the drug budget to take account of the need for the new drugs, so consultants who used them would deprive colleagues of the funding for equally important treatments. The health authority are unmoved by the potentially huge savings in residential care costs. Residential care is paid for by social services, and is not their concern.

'In the next door authority (Kensington, Chelsea and Westminster) people with Alzheimer's disease get the drugs and have a chance of temporary remission to say goodbye to their families, make a will or take a holiday or two. Here in Ealing, Hounslow and Hammersmith we psychiatrists just tell people there's nothing we can do. Like oncologists, we each have to decide whether to say that something can be done but someone is too tight-fisted to let us do it.'

After much pressure from the doctors, the health authority has now proposed that the dementia drugs can be used but on condition that a nurse screens the patients for suitability before prescription and for evidence of improvement after-wards. And they will only pay half the cost of the drugs, with the trust expected to find the other half out of (non) existing funds.

The Government hopes that all this controversy will vanish when the National Institute of Clinical Excellence (NICE) kicks in and tells us all what's worth prescribing and what isn't. However, its early judgements suggest it will err on the side of caution and demand that new drugs have more extensive testing 'in the field' before being widely and fairly available on the NHS. Those lucky enough to live near a hospital carrying out a clinical trial might get a new drug, and those who don't, won't. So just another form of postcode prescribing.

Nobody Loves a Whistleblower

8 June 2000
Letter of the week

Dear Sir,
Thanks for exposing postcode prescribing of dementia drugs at Ealing, Hammersmith and Fulham NHS Trust. On the day of publication, the clinical director was not pleased and reduced one of my colleagues to tears on the assumption that it was she who had spoken to you. More interestingly yet, we have all received a three-line-whip memo

advising us that we have to go to the chief executive's office in order to 'discuss the recent article in *Private Eye* which featured the trust'. It seems that he is determined both to find out who talked to the *Eye* and to give us all a bollocking. We're all a bit shit-scared, and have persuaded the Prof. of Psychiatry to attend and one of my colleagues is taking legal advice. Dr. T. at Ealing is so scared he shuts his doors and windows before he talks on the phone . . .

Whitewash of the Week

The Ritchie Report into the gynaecological devastation caused by Rodney 'The Butcher' Ledward is the usual old bollocks. Something must be done . . . lessons will be learned . . . blah de blah de blah. The failings have been loosely directed at managers, but none have been called to account, disciplined or asked to go on retraining. Why did the health authority not act, having paid out for Ledward's failed surgery on at least nineteen occasions between 1980 and 1994? Why was he not sacked, rather than allowed to retire and keep his full pension? And how did he become a consultant in the first place?

As a Professor of Obstetrics who worked with Ledward as a junior doctor put it: 'He was a cowboy even then. The worst I've ever come across in my career. Whoever gave him good references and supported his consultant appointment perjured their soul to the devil and will carry their consequences to the grave.' Alas, surgeons do not have to perform a practical at interviews but someone, somewhere must have written Rodney sparkling references. I think we should be told who.

Another GMC Cockup

11 August 2000

Hot on the heels of Rodney Ledward is rogue gynaecologist Richard 'Struck Off in Canada in 1985 but fit to practise in the UK' Neale. The GMC's defence for not protecting patients from his dreadful surgery is that it is only allowed by law to take the criminal convictions of overseas doctors into account when considering an application to practise in the UK.

Neale was already working in the Friarage Hospital in Northallerton, North Yorkshire when he was erased from the Canadian register. The GMC was informed of this by the Canadian panel, and by Neale's former colleague and friend Dr Andrew Sear: 'The GMC basically told me that what a doctor did in another country was no concern of theirs.'

A string of senior NHS doctors somehow contrived to give Neale excellent references for his clinical care. So why then did the GMC belatedly conclude that he botched scores of operations, left women haemorrhaging, performed surgery without consent and carried out substandard work?

The secretive self-regulation of doctors is still a sham. The Government and GMC have nothing in place to stop another Bristol, Ledward or Neale from recurring. As Richard Neale said in his final plea to the GMC:

'So what am I? A surgeon who had his best interests at heart.'

'Would you read that again please?'

'So what am I? A surgeon who had his best interests at heart . . .'

'Can I just pause? I asked you twice to read the first sentence again. In my copy it says, "A surgeon who had his patients' best interests at heart."'

'What did I say?'

'Your best interests.'

'I beg your pardon, a Freudian slip.'

An Easy Target

27 September 2000

Macho health secretary Alan Milburn had a tough choice in deciding whom to abolish in his National Plan for the NHS. Would he take on the might of the medical profession and finally put the self-serving, incompetent General Medical Council out of its misery? Or would he piss all over Community Health Councils, the single source of independent, patient-led, local scrutiny of the NHS? Not wishing to duck a difficult decision, Milburn never once discussed the option of abolishing CHCs with their national association prior to burying their abolition in the back end of his Plan. Of the 600 members now facing redundancy, many only found out by logging on to the DoH website.

Milburn has since been keen to lay into his soft target, describing CHCs as 'an outdated model that no-one believes in any more' and 'dinosaurs without relevance to the modern NHS'. So why did a poll of nearly 2,000 readers of the *Health Service Journal* (generally people who manage the NHS and know more about it than Milburn) find 88% in favour of keeping them? Probably because they don't trust the Government to come up with anything better. Milburn's suggested replacement is another ridiculous acronym – PALS (patient advice and liaison service) in every hospital, and a duty for local government to scrutinise local NHS changes. So much for independence.

In fact, CHCs were established by statute in 1974 to have scrutiny and inspection roles in addition to patient advocacy. Despite pitiful funding (the average CHC in England has a disposable budget of £20,000 a year), they have forced through many local improvements and caused successive governments embarrassment with their national surveys of the conditions, waiting times and trolley-stops in hospitals. Their major problem is a lack of teeth – any concerns they raise can be easily steamrollered by government.

Instead of abolishing England's 182 CHCs, Milburn would be better advised to tap into their local knowledge to improve accountability in the NHS. Earlier this year, the national association for CHCs set up an independent commission chaired by Will Hutton which found the NHS to be 'woefully unaccountable'. One suggested solution – to make the NHS a semi-independent public corporation with constitutional independence from politicians – may have been too much for the meddling, ambitious Milburn. Closing down CHCs will make his life easier but the NHS even less accountable.

Waiting for the President

17 September 2000

In June 1999 I received anonymous concerns about the standard of heart surgery at the Brompton Hospital in London. Instead of publishing them, I faxed them back to the chief executive, who instigated a prompt and thorough inquiry. I also sent them to Sir Donald Irvine, president of the GMC. I did not receive a reply after 56 days. The GMC then drafted a letter to the *Lancet* stating I'd never asked for a response, before retracting it, issuing me with a written apology and advising me not to send mail requiring a swift reply directly to the president.

A Member for Life

29 September 2000

Alan Maynard, director of health policy at the University of York, has written to the *Eye* with his interpretation of how dodgy gynaecologist Richard Neale got away with it for so long: 'It seems that when Northallerton Trust discovered both his awful results in Canada and his incapacity to improve in North Yorkshire, they paid him over £100,000 in 'compensation' and gave him a good reference so he could continue his pain and misery elsewhere. But was NHS management to blame for this?'

Not entirely, argues Maynard, who cites the ridiculous regulations that NHS managers are bound by, and which successive governments have refused to change. At present, a consultant cannot be sacked without 'due cause', and the disciplinary procedure is so protracted that it allows doctors to appeal to the Secretary of State. The doctor may be suspended for years on full pay, leaving no funds for a replacement, while waiting lists rise leaving hospitals facing further penalties for failing to meet government targets. So it's far easier (and cheaper) to let a deviant keep operating.

Maynard also points out that although the GMC is embarrassingly inept at self-regulation, it is the Royal Colleges who are responsible for overseeing training. Ten years ago, when minimally invasive (keyhole) surgery was introduced, training was patchy to non-existent and a great deal of harm was caused by surgeons learning the ropes. And those surgeons found guilty of serious professional misconduct by the GMC (e.g. the Bristol two, Neale, Ledward) don't even have their Royal College affiliations withdrawn. Once a member, always a member – unless you fail to pay the annual subscription (got to keep those wine cellars stocked).

Regulating the NHS

20 October 2000
'When hospitals are fighting each other for survival, it's the ones with the most psychopathic doctors who come out on top.' So said an Oxford surgeon about the downsizing of London's teaching hospitals under the Conservatives. His

observation is perhaps a tad harsh, but the pathological institutional loyalty of doctors is an important barrier to improving the health service. Doctors are chosen for their extreme academic ability, and by their nature are obsessive, compulsive, over-achieving workaholics. You get plenty of hours out of us, provided you leave us alone to build our empires without criticism. Indeed, I've had more scrutiny for writing this column (including six hours in the witness box at a public inquiry) than in thirteen years as a doctor.

This was not a theme explored in Channel 4's *Doctors on Trial* series, which tried to present research on medical errors dating back to 1989 as something new. Doctors are human, they make mistakes and 25,000–40,000 patients a year die in the NHS as a result.

The programmes put this down to faults in 'the system' (of which there are plenty) without questioning the logic of a profession that allows its members to perform life-threatening surgery without ever having to prove they're any good at it. At present, only 17% of hospitals have a strategy in place for continuously monitoring and improving quality. So for most of the hospital service (and pretty much all of general practice) we haven't got a clue if patients are getting an acceptable standard of care or not.

A good start would be routinely collecting outcomes to define safe standards and spot 'statistical outliers' who may not be safe. And we should routinely pick up single medical errors, discuss them and learn from them – and swiftly compensate patients who've been harmed (rather than see everyone's money swallowed up in legal fees).

Body Counts

24 November 2000

Jan Poloniecki, a lecturer in medical statistics at St George's Hospital in London, has spent a lot of time proving that hospitals don't even know what their body count is: 'The mortuary registers in many UK hospitals are still not computerised but are hand-written, and around 20% of deaths are missed in audit systems.... In consequence a typical hospital will every month send out letters to twenty dead patients reminding them of their appointments. Two of these "patients" will have ambulances come round to pick them up. On one occasion, the ambulance and the hearse arrived at the same time.'

Poloniecki's most recent study is to analyse body counts after heart surgery at St George's and St Thomas's Hospitals. Four patients were incorrectly coded as leaving the hospital alive and fewer than 80% of the deaths at St Thomas's made it onto all the departmental databases and the hospital administration system. This in a specialty that is way ahead of the field in data collection. Overall, the hospital mortality statistics submitted across the NHS for the Government's league tables are likely to be very inaccurate and erring on the low side.

The situation at St George's has been improved by installing a computer link from the mortuary to double-check the figures, and taking responsibility for their accuracy locally. In contrast, chief medical officer Liam Donaldson has persuaded the Department of Health to set up a critical-incident register relying on voluntary reporting to a remote central database. This is a further recipe for inaccuracy and suggests the exercise is little more than cosmetic. Only the statutory reporting of errors and near misses to a locally administered register with good statistical input is likely to achieve anything meaningful that can then be compared to other hospitals.

This lack of meaningful information is likely to plague the

Commission for Health Improvement (CHI) as it endeavours to ensure high-quality care in the NHS. Its first two high-profile 'hits' were at the now closed Garlands Hospital, Carlisle, where staff had been beating up patients for years and it was well known in-house, and at Prince Philip Hospital, Llanelli where a pensioner had a wrong kidney removed many months ago. Whether CHI's ground-breaking recommendations (e.g. mark X-rays to show which is right and which is left, listen to the medical student when he tells you you're operating on the wrong kidney) will make any difference remains to be seen.

A third investigation – at the Oxford Heart Centre – was commissioned by the NHS Executive South East. It made some headline-grabbing assertions about the unit ('on its knees and riven by internal conflict') but was almost devoid of statistical analysis. The Oxford Heart Centre has already been fingered in the Bristol inquiry for failing to submit results to the Society of Cardiothoracic Surgeons' register. Neither has it bothered to submit results to the national database, leaving it very vulnerable to criticism.

Brain Surgery Secrecy

6 December 2000

Two patients have contacted the *Eye* having suffered complications after brain surgery in Bristol. Both had pituitary tumours removed by the same surgeon at Frenchay Hospital, part of the North Bristol NHS Trust, and both now have permanent damage to their visual fields. They want to know if they were just unlucky or whether they got a sub standard service. Having met with the usual wall of secrecy from the NHS, they're now asking other patients who may have suffered similar complications to contact them via the *Eye*.

Pituitary surgery needs to be done by specialists. In the *BMJ*

(May 8, 1999), John S Bevan, a consultant endocrinologist at Aberdeen Royal Infirmary, stressed the importance of treatment by specialist multidisciplinary teams in regional centres who all comply with best practice, rather than the hugely variable preparation and monitoring of patients that currently occurs: 'Pituitary surgery should always be performed by a specialist surgeon. This is particularly important for patients with hormonally-active tumours where surgical skill is a critical determinant of success.'

In September 1999, another paper looked at surgery for pituitary tumours that cause acromegaly and found that of 73 patients operated on by nine surgeons in Manchester, fewer than 20% had a successful outcome. In Birmingham, where eight surgeons operated, the success rate was 33%. When a single surgeon took over, the success rate doubled to 66%. In Oxford, Newcastle and Bart's, the operations are also done by a single surgeon and the success rate ranges from 42 to 56%.

This is clearly bad luck for the patients who got a surgeon who only did the operation occasionally, but – as with most of medicine – incompetence is near impossible to prove. The same is likely to be true of the situation in Bristol. In July 1999, I received concerns raised by a consultant about the standard of pituitary surgery there. The consultant described himself as 'really worried' and said of one surgeon: 'we have done our best to steer pituitary patients away from him . . . the life of one of my patients has been all but ruined by a dramatic reduction in his visual field after surgery.'

I contacted the General Medical Council, the Royal College of Surgeons and the chief executive of North Bristol NHS Trust and asked that the matter be investigated. Sixteen months later and I've been told that an internal audit has found no statistical difference in the outcomes from the two surgeons, and their results are comparable to elsewhere in the UK. However, none of the audit has been made public and there is still no prospective national database of pituitary surgery in the UK to compare the results of different centres. As with most complex surgery, neurosurgeons are allowed to delve into brains without having to prove they're any good at it.

Meanwhile, the consultant who raised concerns suffered a fair degree of professional vilification, including a call for his sacking from a board member of NBNT for daring to question the quality of the service. He now doubts he would whistleblow again and says; 'I have retired hurt from pituitary politics. . . . I just see the damage.'

A Day Out in Bristol

18 December 2000

I got a warm welcome when I accompanied a relative for heart surgery at the Bristol Royal Infirmary last month. As one member of staff remarked to the professor of surgery, 'You know who that is, don't you? You'd better not fuck this one up.' Fortunately, the standards of angiography and surgery were superb and any lingering doubts about the expertise of the staff were dispelled by the unit's excellent prospective audit, which is still the only one in the UK to be published on the internet.

However, the surroundings left a little to be desired. The angiography suite is in a new building on one side of the road and has a spanking new ward nearby that's ideal for patients to recuperate in and be closely watched, in case an artery blocks off suddenly (a recognised complication). Alas, the ward has been allocated to Care of the Elderly, which means that following angiography, patients have to go three floors down and into a dark tunnel under the road (known locally as 'the dungeon') and up again to recover on the less than salubrious Ward 20. If their heart stops suddenly, then it's back down to the dungeon and in the lift, with staff furiously pummelling the chest in the hope they can make it back to the angiography suite. The fact that the management have not grasped the idiocy of this situation is symptomatic of their general disinterest in improving the service.

Elsewhere, there are beds in corridors, patients on chairs praying for a bed, and patients in beds who've been waiting for surgery for months. Their plight was bravely championed by Peter Wilde, radiologist and director of cardiothoracic services for the United Bristol Healthcare NHS Trust, who made Tony Blair look like a floundering guppy during the televised debate into the state of the NHS held at St Thomas's in March. He surprised Blair with evidence of big regional differences in funding: 'We have only half the national level of funding for heart surgery, and we have 700 patients on our waiting lists, of which 100 have been waiting for more than a year for open-heart surgery. In the last six months twenty patients have died while waiting for this surgery. We fall not 5% or 3% below the national average; we fall 45% below. We are being committed to waiting-list targets, and yet 70% of our patients are also urgent and need to be operated on immediately.'

The Government has now bunged a few extra million Bristol's way to gloss over the shortcomings in angiography resources, but it has come too late for Wilde, who has resigned his management position in despair. Other consultants talk not just of the lack of central funding, but of the managerial apathy which continually undermines the work of the unit and prevents it from becoming truly innovative.

Jaws Bites Back

4 January 2001
Following the damning external review into the Oxford Heart Centre, *Eye* reader W F Cooke has written to the John Radcliffe

Hospital to demand a refund for the quadruple bypass he was forced to pay for privately. Mr Cooke forked out £10,000 of his own money for a bypass in 1997, having been told that the NHS waiting list was at least twelve months. Mr Cooke chose to use half of his retirement lump sum rather than risk dying on the list, and is particularly angry that the lack of effective management in Oxford during that period led to a fall in the annual number of heart operations from 1,400 to 800, and a 30% increase in those waiting at least nine months for urgent surgery. The report also found that the process of allocation of patients for operations was 'chaotic' and that 'private patients always appear to be first on the list'. Now why's that then?

A surgical unit has to be in pretty dire straits before the Royal College of Surgeons does anything, but it was forced to withdraw training recognition from Oxford, a situation unparalleled in the history of heart surgery (even the Bristol unit managed to sail through its RCS inspections during its times of crisis). However, Oxford surgeon Stephen Westaby has been quick to defend the unit's record in a letter to *The Times*, citing the £1.5 million raised privately for trials into an artificial heart, which earned him plenty of Brownie points in the Trust. On the subject of surgical training, he gives a more telling insight in a new book, *Succeeding in Hospital Medicine: The Experts Share Their Secrets* (Health Press).

'I was captain of cricket and rugby ... and my single-mindedness was recognised with the award of "Student Most Likely to Succeed" in 1972. . . . During my surgical training in Cambridge, I was nicknamed "Jaws" and operated on anything and everything day and night. . . . The heart is unforgiving and should never be the first target organ for a trainee surgeon. . . . Britain's lead in cardiac surgery began to dwindle rapidly as private practice took surgeons out of NHS hospitals. . . . In 1986, at the age of 37, I was appointed consultant to the new regional cardiothoracic unit in Oxford. This presented the unique opportunity for a new direction in cardiac surgery as there were no senior colleagues. Within a few years, the number of operations increased from 150 to 1,800 patients a year.' So where did it all go wrong?

Westaby was quick to point out in *The Times* that his unit has 'the lowest death rate in the world for dissected aorta', but ignores the fact that – nearly six years after the Bristol tragedy – Oxford still can't be bothered to submit figures to the national database. No such database exists yet for child heart surgery, because no-one has agreed a process of risk-stratification for children that would compensate surgeons doing harder operations.

However, one senior heart surgeon has told me that this is no reason for a unit not to publish its figures: 'All the child heart surgery units around the UK treat roughly comparable groups of children. There are no genetic clusters of particular forms of congenital heart disease in the UK that I am aware of, and so there really is no excuse not to come clean about your figures. If your unit's mortality is around 3–6% then you have nothing to worry about, but if it's up above 10%, that centre needs urgent investigation, risk-stratification or not. At present, the system is still geared to protecting doctors' reputations rather than protecting patients from unnecessary harm.'

Spot the GP

29 March 2001

The Government's promise of 2,000 extra GPs as soon as possible seems to be falling on deaf ears, at least in Wales. Not a single doctor has applied for the Swansea GP training scheme, due to start in August, and the Bridgend scheme has yet to find 'a single suitable applicant'. The health minister John Denham recently tried to reassure GPs at the NHS Alliance spring conference that the NHS Plan 'should not mean a single doctor will have to work harder. If it does, then we have failed.' No GP agreed, and all present claimed to be working much harder.

Neither were they impressed by Alan Milburn's offer of a £10,000 'Golden Goodbye' for any GP foolish enough to hang on to 65. According to actuarial statistics, GPs who work till 65 tend to die by 68, whereas those who get out before 60 live, on average, to 78. So bribing clapped-out doctors to stay behind the wheel another five years actually saves the Treasury a small fortune in pensions.

One Sick Doctor

Hospital doctors too seem to be cracking under the strain. A diagnostic radiologist ('name and address supplied') has written the following letter to the trade magazine *Hospital Doctor*: 'There are a substantial number of patients out there who are unutterably execrable. . . . They are in the main at worst trivially unwell. They need no attention (apart from a good slapping) but insist on being seen. . . . I can only imagine the horror of seeing a waiting room full of these churls and ingrates all bleating louder than sheep, knowing that there is damn-all wrong with them. I have a mental image of revenge – turning to a most loathsome specimen, smiling thinly while declaring, "You've got cancer you bastard – die soon."' Clearly the GMC's insistence that all doctors 'make patients their first concern' has a little way to go.

Lots of Sick Doctors

The Government's National Clinical Assessment Authority (NCAA) was launched this month to help identify (and retrain) 'underachieving doctors'. The NCAA claims that it will give doctors a 'fairer and faster' resolution of complaints against them but there are already 250 doctors on suspension in the UK so it will have its work cut out. Even the GMC accepts that there could be 13,000 drug- or alcohol-dependent doctors out there, waiting to be discovered. The BMA does not trust the Government to help medical addicts and if they were all suspended the NHS would fall to pieces. But the profession's own record in this area is pretty lamentable.

BMA ethics committee member Dr Michael Wilks has been lobbying hard to get the BMA to take addiction seriously, with little progress: 'I have had little success in getting the BMA, the GMC, Royal Colleges and medical defence bodies to invest in a scheme similar to the American "Impaired Physicians' Program". In the USA and Canada, 85–90% of addicted doctors are sober and in work five years after treatment. The Priory would kill for that sort of result. There is also evidence from California that recovering doctors are sued less often than the rest.'

Given that we have so few doctors in the UK, it seems absurd that such a programme isn't up and running in the UK. Perhaps the only hope is for addicted doctors who fall foul of the NCAA to cancel their subscriptions to the BMA and Royal Colleges until they act. If the stocks in the wine cellar start to fall, they'll soon take an interest.

Trust Me, I'm a Locum

11 May 2001
The failure of Labour to produce any tangible improvement in the quality of NHS care over its first term in office is exemplified by its inability to protect patients from substandard locums. The NHS employs over 3,500 locum doctors a day to fill huge gaps in the service and although most probably are competent, no effective checks are in place to ensure this.

Earlier this month the Commission for Health Improvement (CHI), reported on Dr James Elwood, a 78-year-old pathologist allegedly responsible for over 215 errors and at least seven cases of 'serious harm' between 1994 and 2000. For some reason, the Government's tough new independent watchdog 'did not set out to assess his competence and has no evidence either way.' And neither will the GMC act, since he has voluntarily removed himself from the medical register. But CHI's director Peter Homa spotted that Swindon and Marlborough Trust's failure to check where he had worked before and whether he was up to the job was 'shocking'. And that 'all over the country trusts continue to appoint locum doctors without proper checks and then fail to monitor their performance.'

Haven't we heard this somewhere before? In 1994, Sir Robert Kilpatrick, then president of the GMC, stressed the obligation of doctors to monitor their colleagues: 'At all times patient safety must take precedence over all other concerns, including understandable reticence to bring a colleague's career into question.' This after a consultant had failed to investigate complaints that a locum anaesthetist, Dr Behrooz Irani, was endangering patients. Dr Irani left a 33-year-old man seriously brain-damaged and in a persistent vegetative state, nearly repeated the error six months later, and had previously been suspended by the GMC for stealing two ventilators. But he still got work in East Yorkshire because they were so short of staff.

Following this, Chief Medical Officer Kenneth Calman set up a working party to investigate the system of appointing locums. It reported in 1995, recommending tighter scrutiny for hospital locums and the setting up of a central database of doctors who are found to be unsatisfactory. A year later, these proposals were still 'under review' when the NHS Executive promised 'more robust standards' when appointing locums after investigations into 531 diagnostic errors by Dr Samuel Kiberu, a locum consultant pathologist, at two hospitals in Grantham and

Bassetlaw. The importance of closer scrutiny was also stressed by the edentulous Royal College of Pathologists.

After another year of feverish inactivity, youthful health minister Alan Milburn entered the locum fray in 1997, announcing a 'crackdown on locum doctors. The existing rules governing locum doctors are inadequate. In future all locum doctors will be screened to weed out those who are a danger to patients.' This followed a serious sexual assault on a child patient by a locum surgeon. Two years of pointless rubber-stamping later and the (1999) Audit Commission was unimpressed: 'Although there have been several reports suggesting that the recruitment and induction procedures for locum doctors need to be improved, there is little evidence of this having happened ... professional qualifications, past criminal convictions, and references are still often not checked. Consultants admitted that they often don't even meet the locum.'

In April 2001, the Audit Commission noted little improvement on the quality control of locums in Wales, and in general practice several large studies have found that qualifications, references and past convictions are often not checked prior to employment. This is not surprising to anyone from Bradford, where bogus doctor Mohamed Saaed 'practised' for 30 years. He prescribed creosote for a sore throat, shampoo for conjunctivitis and survived two competency checks from real GPs before his family shopped him.

The current chief medical officer Liam Donaldson has promised to cut down on medical errors with a new central database and his ironically entitled project *An Organisation with a Memory*. The CHI too has implored the Department of Health to 'make proper checks on locums'. And Alan Milburn has promised the *News of the World*: 'My alarm bells will trap dodgy docs' (11 June 2000). But back on earth the NHS is desperately short-staffed and locums often end up working in appalling conditions. The fact that the NHS needed to employ

Elwood, a 78-year-old pathologist, is bad enough, but he was working in sub standard accommodation using outdated equipment rejected by other doctors and with a disproportionately high workload. Welcome to Labour's 'First Class NHS ... where there is no room for second best'.

The Bristol Inquiry Finally Reports

20 July 2001

'There are no winners in Bristol. We are all losers.' So said charity director and parent Maria Shortis when the report was finally published last week. But perhaps the biggest losers are the surviving children left permanently brain-damaged by heart surgery. As no unit in the country has kept reliable data on morbidity (i.e. damage short of death), Kennedy was not able to offer any judgement as to whether this was excessive in Bristol compared to an average unit over the eleven years under study. These children have already been forgotten once, by the earlier GMC inquiry, and are offensively recorded in the hospital statistics as 'successes' because they were still alive 30 days post operation.

There are at least 30 such children who need constant care and whose parents face a living hell. Many have a normal life expectancy but because proving clinical negligence is so difficult, they may never receive compensation unless Milburn acts swiftly on Kennedy's suggestion to introduce retrospective no-blame compensation as a gesture of goodwill.

However, ditching negligence litigation before proper mechanisms of accountability are in place in the NHS (which clearly aren't yet), could make it harder to uncover the other Bristol-type disasters that Kennedy believes we can't discount. Were it not for the tenacity of lawyers such as Laurence Vick in the Bristol case, the trust might never have handed over the surgeons' logbooks that helped prove the care was so inadequate.

Another loser in Bristol is the courageous paediatric heart surgeon Ash Pawade, who took over in 1995 when Wisheart and Dhasmana finally threw in the scalpel. Very few, if any, other heart surgeons would have entered such a stressful environment. And yet, immediately, his expertise shone through, despite suffering the same substandard working conditions and split sites as the previous incumbents. While they lost nine out of thirteen babies to the switch operation, he and his colleagues have now performed the operation over 70 times without a single fatality.

The reward for such incredible results should surely be a top merit award, particularly since Wisheart retired with the top A+ grade for services to the profession. Yet despite the promises of health secretaries Dobson and Milburn that these archaic awards would be overhauled to ensure the money goes to those who best serve patients, Pawade has been repeatedly overlooked, along with the equally gifted and progressive adult surgeon Gianni Angelini. Both have done more than anyone to put heart surgery back on the map in Bristol but both, like anaesthetist Steve Bolsin before them, are 'outsiders'. Clearly the club culture is alive and kicking in Bristol and they aren't members.

Outside Bristol, which was rightly praised by Kennedy for publishing its results, the other twelve heart surgery units were also losers for failing to take the opportunity to demonstrate their competence to the public. British Paediatric Cardiac Association president Bob Anderson deserves credit for persuading all the units to at least collect data for the year up to April 2001, which has apparently found that there are no statistically significant poor performers and overall results that are as good as any in the world. However, he wasn't able to release the audit into the public domain because the units hadn't all agreed to it. So we just have to take it on blind trust again. Surely if the information is good enough to reassure us that child heart surgery disasters are no longer occurring, it's good enough for individual units to publish?

Whose Embryo Is It Anyway?

3 August 2001

Who regulates the Human Fertilisation and Embryology Authority? The HFEA is a statutory body set up in 1991 to ensure all UK treatment clinics offering IVF, donor insemination (DI) or the storage of eggs, sperm and embryos conform to acceptable standards – a task which many specialists believe it has neither the resources nor expertise to do. However, it is its further ethical role, to license and monitor human embryo research, that has attracted the most criticism.

The HFEA is a quango of 21 government-appointed members, with more than half 'coming from disciplines other than medicine or human-embryo research.' This is apparently to ensure 'a wide spectrum of interests and views' but in effect has made it excessively restrictive to new technology. Its 'successful judgements' include holding up the development of a valuable sperm injection technique, ISCI, by three to five years compared to the rest of Europe. It also made an absurd ruling that human eggs could be frozen but not thawed for therapeutic purposes, a decision they have now mercifully reversed but not before a patient was subjected to a horrendous amount of media attention and stress. And sperm imports to the UK were also held up for two years.

The latest delaying tactic has been to prevent IVF clinics from screening embryos prior to implantation, which improves pregnancy rates by 10% and reduces miscarriages by half. This is especially important because overall success rates for IVF are never more than 20% and older women have far more chance of producing embryos with too many or too few chromosomes. As with all screening, there is a risk of misdiagnosis but there is also the potential to avoid some extremely disabling and rapidly fatal diseases. In January, James Yeandel of the HFEA gave the stock answer: 'We won't be rushed, or bulldozed or forced into action by clinicians. We are here to make sure science does not move ahead faster than the public wants.'

All new innovation involves some risk, but the net effect of the HFEA's policy has been to drive many of the UK's best fertility researchers abroad to Europe and the USA, where they develop innovative treatments which then only become available to UK patients many years later. The HFEA recently produced a press release celebrating the 50,000 babies born to IVF treatment since UK scientists successfully pioneered the technique in 1978, but had the HFEA been in existence then, we'd still be waiting for the first birth.

Alan and Louise Masterton have four sons and lost their only daughter in a bonfire accident. They applied to the HFEA last year for permission to screen and implant embryos of a chosen sex in the very specific and rare instance where a couple have lost a child of one sex and already have at least one child of the other sex. In the Mastertons' case, this would not involve the death of any male embryos, which they would donate to another couple. They have also undergone extensive psychological testing to ensure, as far as is possible, that their decision would not have a detrimental effect on existing family members.

The application was rejected by the HFEA in a manner described by Alan Masterton as 'obstinate and uncaring'. In a society that allows mass abortion for purely psychological reasons, it seems bizarre that you can't create a child of a given sex for far more compelling psychological reasons. And Ruth

Deech, chairman of the HFEA, appeared to show a complete misunderstanding of their application when questioned on BBC World's *HARDtalk* programme: 'It is not ethical to throw away the boy embryos and only use the girls' – something the Mastertons have never suggested. 'It's also wrong to value one gender above the other, you start there and you'll have people saying for all sorts of frivolous reasons they want a boy, not a girl.' Yet there is nothing remotely frivolous in the Mastertons' very specific appeal.

The ultimate fallback for the HFEA is to claim they are mirroring public opinion, but in the case of the gender-selection argument, this is based on an outdated public survey gathered in 1991–92. When the Mastertons put their specific request to the public on BBC online, STV and Ceefax, they received support of 71%, 60% and 47%. These are hardly random samples, but neither was the HFEA's. It's time the HFEA experienced some regulation itself.

More Broken Hearts

13 September 2001

The supposedly independent Commission for Health Improvement, suspiciously quiet during the election run-up, has now stirred itself into action with its report into heart and lung transplant failings at London's St George's Hospital between December 1999 and September 2000, when eight out eleven patients died within 90 days of heart transplant. Transplant units are supposed to achieve an 80% survival rate one year after operation. CHI chief executive Peter Homa concluded: 'The wrong patients were given the wrong operations by a team whose leadership had broken down and who failed to follow their own rules about which patients should receive heart transplants. No one doctor or manager is responsible for this, but many people in many roles share an accountability for what happened.'

This new 'no individual blame' approach is in stark contrast to the Bristol tragedy, but is it any more likely to prevent repetition? The fact that it took the CHI almost a year to reach its conclusions makes a mockery of Labour's promise of a rapid response to NHS failings. The doctors as a whole were praised for the speed with which the problem was addressed, but why did it take eight deaths? Statistically it can be hard to differentiate between an unlucky run and avoidable tragedy until you notch up a few failures, but why was no-one analysing each individual case? Surely just one wrong patient given the wrong operation should be enough to send the balloon up?

As soon as a patient died, it appears everyone lost interest. The CHI found that very few deaths were referred for postmortem and the few that were done were not always adequate. Little effort was made to understand why patients were dying in order to prevent recurrence. The unit was run down and dirty, there was a lack of effective clinical leadership, the chief executive and clinical director were kept in the dark until well after the problem was spotted, patient records weren't kept properly, the unit's own criteria for transplants were ignored and there was no 24-hour cover for transplant co-ordination. These failings alone should have debarred the hospital from conducting heart transplants without waiting for the results. But only the NHS could let leaderless surgeons perform the most complex surgery in a crumbling shit-hole.

Turning Over Stones

28 September 2001
Pity Peter Homa, the beleaguered chief executive of the CHI. Homa took up office preaching collaboration with NHS staff

('you can't do improvement to people, you have to help them to do it') and reassuring hospitals and GPs that they had 'nothing to fear' from a CHI inspection. But a colleague who met up with him recently observed how distressed and surprised he was by the appalling standards of care in the NHS.

The CHI's first report, nearly a year ago, was a very retrospective look at the long-standing abuse of elderly mental health patients at North Lakeland Trust, and was bound to be 'a hard-hitting attack on management failings'. Its second, into how the wrong kidney was removed from a patient at the Prince Philip Hospital, Llanelli, has led to the arrest of a surgeon on manslaughter charges (so nothing to fear there, then). But Homa was upbeat a year ago: 'These are exceptional cases . . .'

Alas, after a couple of positive reports and a pre-election lull in activity, the CHI's latest four reports have each picked up the tag of 'most damning yet'. The 'catalogue of failures' at Epsom and St Helier NHS Trust, the Loughborough GP who molested male patients unchallenged for years, the heart-transplant patients at St George's who 'need not have died' and, most recently, the report into the University Hospitals of Coventry and Warwickshire where Homa struggled to find a single positive thing to say.

A trend seems to be appearing here that even Alan Milburn can spot, but the solution may be a long time coming. Bristol inquiry chairman Ian Kennedy complained that the NHS has been 'littered' with previous inquiries that were 'consigned to gather dust on shelves.' Yet many of them made precisely the same criticisms of the structure, organisation and resourcing of the NHS that Homa and Kennedy are also making.

In 1965, a letter to *The Times* complained about the shocking treatment of 'geriatric patients in mental hospitals' and the casual attitude of the Ministry of Health in dealing with these problems. Shades of North Lakeland over 30 years later. In 1967, an investigation called *Sans Everything* concluded that the NHS hierarchy denies problems and dismisses complaints as unfounded, even when supported by strong evidence. There is a tendency to lie low and hope the criticism will fade. And complainants are discredited and victimised. This is as good a summary of the Bristol inquiry as you could find.

Joan Higgins, professor of Health Policy at Manchester University, has analysed the dozens of NHS inquiries and found that the same issues keep recurring. Services working in isolation with inadequate leadership, no clear systems for quality of care and accountability, poor communication and complete disempowerment of staff and patients. Labour have at least documented these problems and proposed mechanisms such as clinical governance to address them, but those now charged with scrutinising the NHS are amazed how services can have been left so long to get so poor. Bristol chairman Ian Kennedy was 'outraged' at the patchy provision of children's services.

Those who work inside the NHS just get desensitised to it all. The DoH gets frustrated at the 'resistance to change' in the NHS, but with burn-out and depression affecting around 20% of the NHS workforce it's hard to see where the change is going to come from. Staff recruitment is as dire as ever. At Hinchingbrooke Hospital in Huntingdon, concerns about the danger caused by the lack of experienced staff on the labour ward were raised two years ago, but despite an inquiry recommending the recruitment of ten more G-grade midwives, none have yet been recruited. Some of the best midwives have left, the director of midwifery has gone off sick, none of the junior doctors are career obstetricians and only three of the five consultants are pulling their weight. So the existing midwives are flying by the seats of their pants. Hardly a service built around safety.

Scant Reward

21 November 2001

Staff in the department of cardiac surgery at the Bristol Royal Infirmary hoped that the table-topping results in last week's Dr Foster Beezer Homes Opal Fruit League Table would lead to enough funding to get them out of their grossly cramped and unsuitable premises and into a spanking-new heart centre. Alas, the Department of Health has passed over the idea of relocation in Bristol, and the unit will just get a small slice of the £300 million Mr Milburn has taken away from somewhere else in the NHS to tinker with its waiting lists.

Mr Milburn knows a thing or two about waiting. On July 18, he gave his initial thoughts on the Bristol inquiry and announced: 'Today we are publishing information for patients, and specifically for parents, about the questions they should ask before consenting to treatment for themselves or their children.' Four months later and the questions haven't been released.

Why Doctors Still Make Mistakes

17 December 2001

The Audit Commission's finding that the number of deaths due to drug errors has increased fivefold in the last ten years is no surprise to those who work in the NHS, but the Department of Health's target to reduce these by 40% by 2005 seems a little optimistic. The NHS itself is now one of the leading causes of premature death and disease in this country, with 25,000–40,000 deaths and half-a-million injuries caused each year by preventable errors alone. Labour has decided that promoting a 'no blame' culture will encourage staff to come forward and admit to cockups, enabling swift action to prevent recurrence. But most doctors and nurses still believe that they'll be named and shamed if they own up to anything, as the experience of Andrew Hobart suggests.

Last year Mr Hobart, a newly appointed consultant in accident and emergency medicine at London's Newnham Hospital, turned the wrong knob on an anaesthetic machine and delivered nitrous oxide to the lungs of a three-year-old girl, rather than oxygen. The girl, Najiyah Hussain, died. The anaesthetic machine in question should have been put out of service years ago because such a fatal error is so easy to make under pressure (and has been made before). But obsolete machines get palmed off on casualty departments where no-one would ever need to use nitrous oxide anyway. It's courting disaster, and any doctor could have made that mistake.

An inquiry reached a similar conclusion, recognised Hobart's commitment and compassion and recommended he be allowed to return to work under supervision. So far, so good for the new no-blame culture. However, the *Daily Mirror* has since reported Hobart to the General Medical Council, who are obliged to investigate further, and the Crown Prosecution Service is waiting in the wings to make everyone suffer a lot more. Clearly Hobart's distress cannot compare to that of the Hussains, but if all the doctors who make fatal cockups each year are hung out to dry, the NHS will collapse.

Nod Off and Die

Falling asleep at the wheel kills more people than drink-driving and is particularly common amongst patients with sleep apnoea. This condition occurs when the airway behind the tongue collapses during sleep and although sufferers wake before suffocation, their disturbed sleep makes them seven times more likely to crash the car. Fortunately, diagnosis and treatment is available at specialist NHS sleep centres. Unfortunately, the waiting lists are horrendously long. In Edinburgh alone, you can wait up to four years for an appointment, although Labour has helpfully divided this up into four blocks of one year so it doesn't breach their waiting-time target.

Anyone for Measles?

6 January 2002
Tony Blair's refusal to disclose details of his son's vaccination status on the grounds that it is a breach of 'the total right to confidentiality of medical records' was not shared by Gordon Brown, who has sanctioned the release of all sorts of information about his daughter Jennifer. We know she suffered from intra-uterine growth restriction, was only 2lbs 4oz at birth, had little surrounding amniotic fluid, was treated with head-box oxygen therapy and ultraviolet light for jaundice and is being fed by an intravenous drip. But we don't know if Leo has had his MMR jab.

Many doctors don't share Blair's reticence (both my children have had both of their MMR jabs) and indeed a recent publication called *Managing Media Hype*, written by a panel of 'practising healthcare professionals with an understanding of the media', advocates personal disclosure as an important strategy for both convincing and alarming patients: 'Tell your patients: "my grandmother got measles as a child and it left her deaf."' Are any of the PM's relatives hearing-impaired through childhood infection? I think we should be told.

Dr Phil's Notes
Cherie Blair was subsequently very forthcoming in her autobiography about where, and under what circumstances, Leo

was conceived (at Balmoral, which always made Tony randy, but without her usual 'contraceptive equipment', which she didn't pack lest it embarrass the butler). The subsequent debate centred on what contraceptive equipment a Catholic mother should use (strictly, just a thermometer for a vague guess at ovulation day, and a tissue to clear up any stringy cervical mucous). But whatever happened to Leo's right to privacy?

Don't Hold Your Breath

18 January 2002

And finally . . . ten years after I suggested heart surgeons should publish their figures in a manner comparable to other units, and two years after suggesting it to the Bristol Public Inquiry, health secretary Alan Milburn has announced that comparative figures for surgeons will be published. But not until 2004. And only death rates up to 30 days. And only adult heart surgeons – although we're working on the rest. Still, it's progress of a sort.

There are legitimate concerns for surgeons and patients, not least the accuracy of the information put on show. The Government's previous performance league tables and those farmed out to private company Dr Foster both fell woefully short of the standards required for fair comparison. Now that individual surgeons and their teams are up for scrutiny, it's vital the Government gets it right or even more of the NHS budget will be frittered away in the courts.

But good-quality information is expensive to gather and analyse, and the Government's 198-page response to the inquiry, *Learning from Bristol*, gives no breakdown of costs at all. Audit information needs to be collected peripherally and analysed centrally by an organisation independent of both the NHS and the Department of Health. But at present, far too much is done by the surgeons themselves, for no money at midnight on the back of an envelope.

Good-quality audit makes the staff up their game and makes the service even better. In Bristol, now one of the most successful units in the UK, audit is published and patients are tracked far longer than 30 days after operation. As Professor Gianni Angelini puts it: 'What's the point of surviving heart surgery if you can't get out of the house with angina a year later?' So his unit collects data on all patients annually. If Bristol can do it now, why can't everyone else?

Epileptic Misfit

1 February 2002

The investigation of consultant paediatrician Dr Andrew Holton by the GMC following the alleged misdiagnosis and over-treatment of children with epilepsy at the Leicester Royal Infirmary should provide some indication as to whether the GMC has matured since the Bristol inquiry. In 1998, the GMC nailed Bristol on two surgeons and a manager when the subsequent public inquiry found systemic failures at every level of the NHS. In retrospect, the GMC's impression that this was just a little local difficulty in Bristol looks laughable.

Dr Holton has already run the media gauntlet in our new 'no blame' culture and he may well have made a number of errors, but his working environment was appalling. He was the sole consultant in neuro-developmental paediatrics and, as with the Bristol surgeons, spent many years asking for (and not receiving) extra staffing and resources. His waiting list, especially for EEG (brain wave) investigation, was ludicrously long and – as with just about every other doctor working in the NHS – there was no-one monitoring his performance and no regular retraining. And although he was working alone, he was certainly not alone in having difficulty with the diagnosis of epilepsy. Across the UK, roughly one in five adults labelled with epilepsy and taking powerful medication for life don't have the disease. And of those who reach the (only) two super-specialist centres in Liverpool and London, the proportion is even higher.

As for treatment of established epilepsy, studies in general practice have shown that many patients are not even seen once a year by their GP, despite picking up repeat prescriptions, and more than 60% could have their treatment improved. So whatever the failings in Leicester, they represent just the tip of a very unpleasant iceberg. As ever in the NHS, the initial barrier to better care is manpower. Recent expert guidelines from the north-west region have recommended that everyone with a possible diagnosis of epilepsy should see a neurologist specialising in the illness within four weeks. The current average waiting time is 28 weeks, and many patients are still being treated by non-specialists and those with inadequate training. At the current level of consultant expansion, the target should be reached by 2019.

A possible solution would be to train specialist GPs to work in community centres to screen all patients with 'fits, faints and funny turns' (over half of whom don't have epilepsy), but this requires both resources and interest from GPs. Epilepsy is extremely stigmatising for patients but viewed by many doctors as dull and boring. None of the twenty specialist registrars currently doing the rounds through the Walton Centre for Neurology and Neurosurgery in Liverpool want to specialise in the disease and most GPs aren't sure who their epileptic patients are and whether they really have epilepsy or not. The disease is just as common as diabetes, but receives a fraction of the media profile and funding because there are no celebrities willing to shout 'I have seizures' from the rooftops.

The situation is particularly desperate in paediatrics, where epilepsy is very hard to diagnose and around a third of children with epilepsy also have learning difficulties such as autism. The need for counselling and support is huge, but rarely are patients followed up into adulthood despite their increased risk of depression and suicide. Whether the GMC focuses on the big picture or a little local difficulty in Leicester remains to be seen. But as elsewhere in the NHS, changes will probably only occur through litigation. Only about a third of women on anti-epileptic medication are adequately counselled and informed about balancing the risks of the drugs and the risks of seizures to the unborn child. Now, a group of them have hired a lawyer and are suing the NHS for lack of informed consent. Queue the floodgates.

Still Safety Last

15 February 2002

The type of anaesthetic machine that contributed to the tragic death of Najiyah Hussain could inadvertently deliver lethal gas mixture without any oxygen at all. In the early eighties the Canadian Society of Anaesthesiologists made it mandatory for all Canadian machines to be equipped with a mechanism to prevent the delivery of so-called hypoxic gas mixtures. However, a recent survey of 51 NHS hospitals found that 27% did not have 'an anti-hypoxia device'. Most of these were located outside theatre suites, in areas where they would be used infrequently or in emergencies, often by staff not aware of the dangers. Across the NHS, around 3,000 such machines are still in operation.

Replacement of all the machines would clearly be expensive, but would be balanced against the huge personal and financial costs of unnecessary death or brain damage. At the very least, the pure nitrous oxide supply which caused Najiyah's death should be replaced with Entonox, the safe 50:50 mixture of nitrous oxide and oxygen given to labouring women. There are dozens more examples of disasters waiting to happen in the NHS when overstretched staff choose the wrong option. Back in 1987, I nearly killed a patient after I flushed her intravenous line with potassium rather than saline, my defence being that the ampoules looked identical and were stored next to each other. Last year, plastic surgeons at Colchester General Hospital mounted the same defence after mixing up a vial of water with the anaesthetic lignocaine.

This drew an unsympathetic response from Professor Wildsmith of Ninewells Hospital in Dundee: 'To blame the labelling is a diversion of personal responsibility that I find unacceptable because even in a busy plastic-surgery unit, the check takes only a second. . . . Don't whinge about the label, read it.' However, with 43% of junior doctors still working above the agreed limit of 56 hours of actual work or 72 hours on-call a week, and most consultants putting in well above their contracted hours, it would be far safer to change the labelling or storage than rely on the 'personal responsibility' of the staff.

Blair's NHS

27 February 2002

Tony Blair was not enamoured of my suggestion that the NHS should be depoliticised (*Your NHS*, BBC1, 20 February) but instead seemed at pains to be held to account for the state of the health service come the next election. Labour will doubtless produce a whole raft of performance indicators over the next few years to 'prove' the NHS is getting better, but with the Prime Minister's job at stake, the pressure will be enormous to buff the statistics and bury bad news.

A more reliable measure of progress would be the views of those working in the NHS. Most of the BBC's medical audience thought it would take at least another ten years of stability and sustained funding for the NHS to be turned round. However, the Government has improved the provision of intensive care beds (the much-publicised shunting of critically ill patients around the country was never a vote-winner) and as it focuses resources on sexy diseases (cancer and heart attacks) it should make some headway.

Alas the equally important Cinderella diseases (e.g. stroke, epilepsy, mental illness, lung disease, dementia, osteoporosis) are likely to remain badly under-resourced. I currently work in genito-urinary medicine (GUM), pretty much bottom of the pile when it comes to celebrity endorsement (herpes ribbon, anyone?) and ministerial interest. The Bristol GUM clinic has been in ludicrously cramped 'temporary accommodation' for ten years. It's built on top of a plague pit, has to be sprayed regularly for fleas and many of the consulting rooms have no natural light or ventilation. On a hot day full of bad odours, it's uninhabitable.

Bristol's facilities are the worst of all the teaching hospitals in the UK, but many district hospitals have equally poor provision. This despite the fact that attendances at GUM clinics have doubled over the last decade to over a million a year in England alone. This has been mirrored by an increase in sexually transmitted infections (STIs). Between 1995 and 2000, STIs increased in the UK by 300,000 with gonorrhoea rising by 31% in the year 2000 alone. In the same year, chlamydia – a major cause of pelvic infection and female infertility – rose by 17% and there were the largest number of new HIV infections since the start of the epidemic.

Unsurprisingly, GUM clinics are struggling to cope. 42% of units are unable to see 'urgent' cases within 24 hours, 77% of 'open access' clinics have to turn patients away and many are resorting to booked clinics only, with 68% offering appointments in a week or more. The Government has promised GP appointments within 48 hours, so why not for GUM? In Labour-speak, the annual gap between capacity and demand in GUM is 100,000 patients, but as none of them are likely to write to *The Times* about the appalling treatment of their warts or syphilis, the Government seems happy to play lip service to STIs.

A further problem is the misconception that if you've got a dose, you'd know about it. At any one time 10% of sexually active people have chlamydia, and one in three will get it during their lifetime. But 80% of women and 50% of men have no symptoms. Screening pilots in the Wirral and Portsmouth have shown clear benefits, but the Government has only committed £47.5 million for its entire sexual-health strategy, just about enough to introduce very limited and patchy screening while leaving nothing for staff recruitment and premises improvement.

The majority of frontline GUM doctoring is done by poorly supervised non-consultant career grade doctors in units often staffed by a single consultant. To cope with the current patient demand the Royal College of Physicians has recommended a consultant expansion of 93% over the next five years and the Association of GUM Departments has estimated that £248 million is needed for capital rebuilding and refurbishment. None of this is likely to happen and many of us will still be working in poorly staffed, over-burdened plague pits come the next election. But at least we'll have Tony Blair to blame.

Dr Phil's Notes

The Bristol sexual health clinic finally relocated in July 2008 to a new building, the Central Health Clinic (appointments 0117 342 6900). I'm reliably informed it has windows that let in fresh air. The centre itself was opened by health minister Dawn Primorolo, who doubtless had a lively discussion with the staff about why Labour has chosen a cheaper cervical cancer vaccine that doesn't protect against genital warts.

Whose Fault Is It Anyway?

27 March 2002

Last year, researchers examining medical records in two London hospitals found that 11% of inpatients experience what is touchingly known as an 'adverse event'. That's either bad luck or a cockup. Rolled out across the NHS, that's 70,000 deaths a year (up 20,000 on the previous best guess) and almost a million injuries in hospitals alone. No-one's got much of a clue what the state of play is in general practice, but suffice it to say that an awful lot of people are killed or injured as a result of coming into contact with the NHS.

This isn't a peculiarly British problem – health systems around the world are waking up to the downside of medical science – but we're extremely bad at acknowledging it. The culture of 'burn the notes, bury the X-rays' and hope the patient dies before he gets to court is still as prevalent as ever. Labour has set up a National Patient Safety Agency to encourage the reporting, and hence learning from, these adverse events and claims to want to encourage 'an open and non-punitive environment.' So why did Alan Milburn ignore the Bristol inquiry's recommendation of no-fault compensation?

As a lawyer, inquiry chairman Ian Kennedy knew perfectly well that the threat of a clinical-negligence claim is the catalyst to manning the barricades and keeping all the bad news under wraps. According to Kennedy, it should be replaced with a new system 'to respond promptly to patients' needs by compensating those who suffer harm arising out treatment from the NHS.' The current system of complaints and negligence claims is so tortuous, prolonged and sadistic that – as one consultant put it – 'you have to be either very rich or very stupid to proceed.' As a result, only a tiny fraction of the million or more harmed by the NHS each year seek redress, and of those only 5% get it. However, this absurdly unjust system has not stopped the NHS paying, or putting aside, £4 billion a year in legal fees.

And it's also very expensive for patients and relatives. Josephine Ocloo is still trying to establish the facts surrounding the death of her daughter Krista in 1996, and the care she received at the Royal Brompton Hospital: 'I wanted to know if anything untoward had happened that should not have. It was very obvious to me early on that she had not been cared for properly and it was a great insult to me that they were not prepared to admit this and to simply tell the truth. If there was negligence, I wanted an open admission and to be offered some form of redress as recognition of the injury. To me this would have constituted accountability, which is vital. It would have shown my daughter counted for something and could not be injured without someone being held to account. I could then come to terms with her death and move on. This would have stopped me from taking legal action.'

Of course none of this happened, and after three inquiries, she brought legal action which last year found that 'the hospital negligently lost one or more opportunities to review Krista's condition,' and this denied Josephine vital information about Krista's risk of sudden death. However, many crucial bits of her medical records have been lost and the judge was unable to conclude that the lack of follow-up and communication was the cause of Krista's death. This is not unusual – causation is near impossible to prove – but as a result, Josephine had costs awarded against her and is now facing financial ruin: 'I won a ruling of negligence but lost my case.'

Jean Brett has been trying to get justice and accountability out of the NHS since 1985, when she was diagnosed as having glaucoma. She subsequently underwent an operation on her right eye at Watford General Hospital. The eye haemorrhaged, and still has a pronounced droop and continues to cause pain. In 1992, she was told an operation would also be required on her left eye. Mrs Brett insisted upon a second opinion. At Moorfields Eye Hospital in London, she learnt that not only was the operation unnecessary, she had never had glaucoma.

She too had devoted much of her time and over £30,000 of her money to getting an explanation, apology and assurance that the work of her consultant has been reviewed to ensure the same mistake has not happened to other patients. As a seventeen-year case history in the failings of the NHS complaints procedure it would take some beating. Indeed, Watford General Hospital has repeatedly encouraged Mrs Brett to take legal action, doubtless hoping she will go broke and give up. In 1999, an independent conciliator instructed the Trust to offer Mrs Brett a solution 'that doesn't make a mockery of her situation.' Three years later, they still haven't. The case continues . . .

Hip Hop

12 April 2002
Would you let someone hammer a great lump of untested metal into the top of your thighbone? It happens every day in the UK. Hip replacements may be one of the success stories of post-war medicine but 10% of them fail to make it to ten years and some pack up much sooner, requiring a much bigger and more painful revision operation. And yet, of the 60-odd different artificial hips used in the NHS and private sector, only a few have good published results over ten years to show that they work. The vast majority are not tested in humans prior to launching and not properly monitored afterwards.

Unsurprisingly, problems aren't picked up until a lot more damage has occurred. Patients given a new hip are reluctant to admit it isn't working and often suffer in silence rather than seek help. Of those that do, 2,000 a year are told their hip prosthesis has failed. The recent recall of the DePuy International prosthesis, because the sterilisation process made it brittle and prone to excessive wear and tear, is one of the few disasters to be picked up. As Professor Chris Bulstrode, an orthopaedic surgeon at Oxford, put it: 'There must be at least twenty hip models currently on the market that are frankly dangerous.'

Back in 1997, I campaigned for a compulsory national register of orthopaedic implants, as in Sweden, to ensure problems were quickly picked up and acted on. Five years down the line, and the rapid-response Department of Health still hasn't decided who should run the registry and even then, reporting won't be mandatory. NICE has at least set targets for hip-prosthesis performance over five and ten years, but unless the audit is properly resourced and mandatory, these will be meaningless.

Most surgeons are too busy cutting waiting lists to monitor their own performance, and in any case, audit should be independently collected to avoid bias. The fact that Labour, for all its bluster about quality, has not even managed to get a compulsory register running to protect patients from unnecessary harm from one of the commonest operations around shows how committed they really are.

Surgeons too are not entirely blameless. As one put it: 'Drug companies are not much different from arms manufacturers. They fly us all out to Florida, pamper us, brainwash us and then get us to use their latest fancy prosthesis.' And once a surgeon's got hooked on a particular gadget, dodgy or not, he tends to stick with it: 'I personally would never use the Ring Hip but I know senior surgeons who still do. It's all they know.'

The absurdity of the current tick-box regulation of prostheses by the Medical Devices Agency (MDA) was exposed by the scandal of the Capital hip, marketed by 3M Healthcare. The MDA can't be bothered to assess products, it just lets manufacturers apply for a stamp of approval from a variety of 'notified bodies' in the EU. Hence, the Capital hip got a meaningless 'CE' mark attesting to its 'non-toxicity' and 'fitness for intended purpose'. It was hammered into 4,700 NHS patients and although the National Audit Office flagged up a possible design fault in 1995, the MDA didn't get round to advising Capital patients to have their hips examined until 1998.

The MDA has introduced a new (voluntary) reporting system for adverse incidents. It's also passing the buck to Europe by asking for legislative changes to ensure better clinical data before a prosthesis is launched, but given that some orthopaedic surgeons have been lobbying for a national register for decades, I wouldn't hold your breath. At present, 70,000 hips are hammered in each year and, isolated enthusiasts aside, we haven't got much of a clue how they're doing until it's too late. When a hip cement called Boneloc was found to have a high failure rate by the Swedish register, it had been used in only fifteen patients. In Britain, it was used on 1,800.

Back in 1993, the *British Medical Journal* warned that the 'fashion trade in joint replacements is costing the health service millions of pounds each year and, even more important, is causing patients unnecessary pain and distress through early failure of unproved implants'. Nearly a decade later, the system of introducing new prostheses is still no more evidence-based than the fashion industry.

So, what should you do if you're waiting for a new hip? The Charnley, Stanmore, Elite and Exeter have good track records. And they wouldn't have stuck any old rubbish in the Queen Mum – she had a Furlong. But the experience of the surgeon is also crucial. A study published in the *Journal of Bone Medicine* in 1996 found that replacements carried out by junior trainees were eleven times more likely to need a revision compared to operations done by consultants. Good luck.

Dr Phil's Notes

There is a national register for orthopaedic implants but it still isn't compulsory. Many NHS orthopods claim that the quality of surgery in some of Labour's new Treatment Centres leaves a lot to be desired, and some have gathered research to prove it. However, their case is weakened by not being able to show that the NHS has got its house in order either. Patients need protecting from sub standard care wherever it occurs.

What, Still No Public Health?

25 April 2002

Hidden away in the Wanless Report is the former bank manager's estimation of the effect of successful reform of the NHS. In 2022, when we may be paying £184 billion a year, the NHS will 'help' to increase life expectancy from 80 to 81.6 years for men and 83.8 to 85.5 years for women. So, a 2% increase over twenty years for all that dosh. This is less to do with the NHS and more to do with the limits of scientific medicine.

In the last century, our life expectancy increased by 30 years but the majority of that was down to improvements in public health. And the biggest challenge facing the UK's health has nothing to do with lack of medicine, but the fact that the rich live ten years longer than the poor. We already have mass involuntary euthanasia – it's called living in the North. A less charitable view is not to blame poverty for the state of our health, but the fact that we've become a population of risk-taking, smoking, alcoholic lard-buckets. Half the NHS budget is deemed to go on illnesses that are (in theory) preventable. Without changing human behaviour, the NHS is doomed.

Alas, the specialty of public health is being decimated by the Labour reforms. District health authorities were abolished in an unseemly rush on April 1, without any clear structure of how to transfer the expertise of public health consultants and non-medical specialists to the new primary care trusts (PCTs), which now control 75% of the budget. Public health resources were already scarce when concentrated in 95 health authorities, but expert teams were built up over years. Now, they're going to be spread across 315 PCTs. In some areas, staff from a single department will now cater for five PCTs. Nearly all their time will be taken up with management and corporate respon-sibilities, with little time left to develop programmes that might improve public health.

A likely outcome is that PCTs will just cherry-pick the aspects of public health they think they need (e.g. running screening programmes) and overlook the rest. But without the public health expertise to help plan how resources can be more fairly allocated, inequalities will increase. Labour's much-trumpeted NHS Cancer Plan and the National Service Frameworks for other diseases also rely heavily on public health consultants to deliver them.

As one public health consultant put it: 'To say that there must always be change and reform is to forget the fundamental public health questions of what is the evidence for it? And what will be the health impact? Right now, there is considerable evidence that successive reorganisations have been wasteful of time, money and people, and have not delivered service improve-ment.' As with all political health reforms, Labour's 'biggest shake-up in 50 years' has largely been made up on the hoof, hasn't been piloted and hence there is no evidence to predict whether it will work. However, it will almost certainly have some unpleasant side effects, particularly for public health.

Dr Phil's Notes

The Wanless Report made some good points but, in politics, the medium is the message, and when it was pointed out that Wanless was also a risk manager for Northern Rock, his star waned and opened up the galaxy for Lord Darzi to save the NHS. Darzi's passage was also eased by the waning of chief medical officer Liam Donaldson, one of the architects of the disastrous and unsafe 'career modernisation' of junior doctors.

Safety, Secrecy and Impotence

20 June 2002

The lack of power and independence of the National Patient Safety Agency (NPSA) was demonstrated again by the suppression of full publication of their pilot study into 'adverse incidents and near misses' at 28 trusts. Whether Milburn's last-minute block was for fear of frightening the horses or because of genuine fears about the accuracy of the data is immaterial. The instinct of the agency itself was to publish in full, until it was ordered not to. Independent, my arse.

And even if it was, it seems unlikely that the current centralised model will do much to instil the essential safety culture at the front line. The most frightening repeated error the NPSA picked up was mixing up identical bags or ampoules of saline (harmless) and potassium chloride (lethal), a cockup which I made some fifteen years ago. The NHS needs an independent safety agency in every region, continuously monitoring and acting on single errors, not waiting until lots of fatalities happen to spot a trend.

Depression Special

31 October 2002

Last month, in case you missed it, was the *Rumble in Reno II*, a tense debate at the University of Nevada about the merits (or otherwise) of antidepressants. The original rumble in 2000 claimed that antidepressants don't work nearly as well as the manufacturers claim, but was hampered by the fact that the researchers didn't have access to all the relevant clinical trials. Drug companies have a habit of suppressing 'disappointing' results, but even on the best evidence, it seemed that many antidepressant medications have trouble out-performing sugar pills.

This perception has now been reinforced by the release of the New Drug Application (NDA) data sets from the US Food and Drug Administration (USFDA) for six newer drugs: fluoxetine (Prozac), sertraline, paroxetine (Seroxat), venlafaxine, nefazodone and citalopram. These were obtained under US Freedom of Information legislation and include all the trials the drug companies would rather keep hidden in the filing cabinet. When all the trials are added together, antidepressants offer a very modest two-point reduction in Hamilton Rating Scale for Depression (HAM-D) scores compared to placebos. This difference is statistically, but not clinically, significant, and has been described by researchers as 'a dirty little secret'.

Indeed, in over half of the clinical trials sponsored by drug companies, they failed to find significant differences between the drug and the placebo. In America at least, most experts accept that the average drug/placebo difference in the treatment of depression is very small, and the debate has moved on to how to interpret it and what to do about it. Most doctors still advocate antidepressants as a frontline treatment for severe depression, but the power of direct-to-consumer advertising in the US is such that thousands of Americans take antidepressants for mild depression or just when they're feeling a bit pissed off.

In October 2001, GlaxoSmithKline ran an advertisement in the *New York Times Magazine* for paroxetine (known as Paxil in the United States). A woman is walking on a crowded street, her face strained, in a crowd otherwise blurred. The headline reads: 'Millions suffer from chronic anxiety. Millions could be helped by

Paxil.' The fact that this advert occurs so soon after September 11 was surely a coincidence, but prescriptions for antidepressants used to treat both depression and anxiety have increased tenfold in the last decade in both the UK and America. We still lag behind the US when it comes to putting toddlers on antidepressants but it's clear that many patients are still being given a false impression of the power of antidepressants, and worse still, many are told that they are 'easy to come off'.

Earlier this year, the USFDA published a new product warning about severe withdrawal symptoms from paroxetine and the International Federation of Pharmaceutical Manufacturers Associations declared GlaxoSmithKline guilty of misleading the public on US television. And they weren't alone. A few years ago, the Defeat Depression campaign of the Royal Colleges of Psychiatrists and General Practitioners advocated educating patients that discontinuing antidepressant treatment 'will not be a problem'. Even when the issue was recognised, an editorial in the *BMJ* minimised the problems.

Now that the truth is out, most patients will still be wedded to their drugs. They aren't nearly as powerful as you were led to believe but if you try to come off them quickly, the side-effects can be worse than the depression. In the long term, psychotherapy seems to be a better bet than drugs for mild to moderate depression, with a better long-term cure rate and fewer side-effects, but it's extremely hard to get on the NHS. Which is why everyone ends up on drugs.

Unsafety First Again

16 December 2002
Labour is still trying to ignore a key recommendation of the Paediatric & Congenital Cardiac Services Review (PCCSR). The PCCSR was set up by the Government to advise on the

implementations of the Bristol Royal Infirmary inquiry. It decided that child heart surgery should be limited to fewer centres of excellence, each performing 300 operations a year. This would centralise expertise, improve working conditions and training, and make audit more meaningful. Although it would have involved considerable upheaval for some members of staff, clinicians were ready to embrace this change.

The Government alas is 'not persuaded', preferring to carry on with the status quo of thirteen surgical units. This is politically much safer, saving the embarrassment of halting surgery in some key constituencies, but risks endorsing the same culture of occasional practice and lack of resources that allowed the Bristol scandal to develop. The issue is not so much the number of cases performed in each unit, but the number of consultants and junior staff required to run a legal rota under the new European working time directive.

By August 1, 2004, no doctor in training must work more than 58 hours a week, falling to 48 hours a week seven years hence. When these trainees become consultants, they must continue with these safe hours restrictions and designated rest periods. To run a legal rota, there will need to be at least four consultants in each unit, and ideally five. Most units currently have only two consultant surgeons, and there aren't enough in training in the UK to allow such a huge expansion and keep all the units open.

Even if surgeons could be tempted in from abroad, the costs would be prohibitive and each individual surgeon would end up doing less than one operation a week. Hardly a recipe for developing expertise. The only sensible solution is to reduce the number of centres performing surgery, which would embarrass politicians and make patients travel further for surgery, safe in the knowledge that they would be treated by someone who had enough supervised training, rest and experience to guarantee competence.

Second Opinion

6 February 2003

Sue Noxall, nursing co-ordinator for the charity Women's Health Concern, has written an illuminating letter to the NHS Executive asking whether NHS patients have a right to a second opinion. Roberta Wallis, from the DoH's Customer Service Centre, replies: 'Patients have no right in law to a second opinion – this has always been the case ... the majority of rights outlined in the Patients Charter are quasi or implied rights and as such are not backed by statute. . . . However, doctors are advised by the GMC that it is good professional practice for patients to be free to seek a second opinion, and this is enshrined in its guidance to doctors.'

In practice, most doctors will arrange a second opinion, although given the difficulty in getting a first one, it leads to lengthy delays. But patients have little protection from those few doctors who refuse to allow another opinion. Countless studies have shown that different doctors make different diagnoses or suggest widely different treatments with any given patient. One study even found that the same doctor treats the same patient differently on different days.[1] If you get into the right part of the NHS first time, you can get truly excellent care. But if you end up in the wrong part with a doctor unaware of his or her limitations and duties, you're stuffed.

Out of Hours

Labour's big selling point for its much-delayed new GP contract is the chance to get out of 24-hour responsibility for patients. This follows the National Survey of GP Opinion,

[1] Do GPs act consistently when they meet the same patient twice? *British Medical Journal* 19 April 1997.

which found an overwhelming desire for GPs to ditch out of hours care (OOH). So who's going to do it? The Government's initial vision was for all OOH calls to be screened by NHS Direct, the nurse-run helpline, with those in need referred to on-call centres, staffed by the odd GP still willing to do OOH and run by the PCT.

Alas, Labour set up NHS Direct as an independent venture, not liaising with the ambulance service and treading on the toes of many GPs who'd effectively sorted out their OOH by forming co-operatives. At their best, co-ops provide an excellent service with most of the GPs working a manageable one or two shifts a month, in addition to their daytime duty. Although NHS Direct was supposed to reduce the pressure on OOH, in reality it has led to a lot of duplication of effort (seriously ill patients having to be triaged twice, first by a nurse and then a GP) and some inappropriate referrals.

Belatedly, the Government has tried to get co-ops and NHS Direct to integrate. Some of these pilots have been successful, but others have taken eons to integrate and co-ops are pulling out. The situation is now so confused that the emergency care tsar, George Alberti, is advising Alan Milburn to cut back the provision of OOH by NHS Direct.

If the resources squandered on NHS Direct had gone into co-ops in the first place, then OOH for much of the country could well have been sorted by now. Alas, many co-op GPs may now decide to opt out of OOH, leaving PCTs over a barrel to private companies who provide on-call services at four times the cost. As for patients, many will just give up and head straight for 999 and casualty.

Dr Phil's Notes

I attended an awards ceremony with the chair of the London Ambulance Service (LAS) who described his organisation, only half jokingly, as the largest GP practice in London. Although the service was set up to deal with emergencies, much of the care they provide would normally be given by GPs, nurses and health visitors. He didn't mind, so long as LAS was paid for it. Paramedics in polyclinics may be the new general practice, for London at least.

On the same table were the chief executive and operations manager of LAS, both wedded to their mobile phones to check if they were meeting the key performance target (75% of calls to serious or life-threatening conditions reached in eight minutes). Usually they do, but not that night (possibly because the best staff were all receiving awards).

The Price of Progress

11 March 2003

The NHS Modernisation Board's annual report has found modest progress in the service, but hardly enough to justify the 21% increase in funding under Labour. Acute activity has increased by just 2% and GP numbers have increased by only 0.7%. So where's all the money going? Expenditure on heart drugs has certainly increased, although the benefits of this are consistently over-emphasised and will only be apparent in the longer term. But it is the culture of excessive target-setting, over-regulation and inspection that is wasting most time and money.

As one nurse puts it: 'I was appointed as a Clinical Nurse Manager (one of Tony Blair's Modern Matrons) at a West Midlands Mental Health NHS Trust in April last year. Since then the Trust has been inspected or assessed by the following bodies: the Commission for Health Improvement, the Mental Health Act Commission, Investors in People, the Clinical Negligence Scheme for Trusts, a Patient Environment Assessment Team and an Improving Working Lives Assessment Team. We spend all our time preparing for, or responding to, such inspections because our bosses' corporate managerialism requires that we chase the next "badge" to put on the Trust letterhead. I shall leave you to imagine who gets the blame when these awards are not achieved and where patient care is on the list of priorities. Please do not print my name.'

It's Good to be in A&E

27 March 2003

More widespread fiddling can be expected in casualty departments as the struggle to meet the '90% of patients to be dealt with within four hours of arrival' target. This rises to 100% next April. Spot-checks started last week and, as usual, trusts have taken on extra staff and even cancelled operations to please the inspectors, before reverting to normal practice when they disappear. Like most Labour targets, it seems like a good idea to the simple-minded, but the reality is far more complicated. As one casualty consultant puts it: 'There is a large group of patients who must spend more than four hours in an Accident and Emergency department, whether they are in an observation ward or the main department. They include patients with asthma who are borderline for admission – 1,500 people die each year from acute asthma.

'Also, some patients with chest pain need to be seen eight to twelve hours after the pain started to do a test that determines whether the pain has come from the heart. The frail and elderly who present late in the evening and live on their own, whose apparent illness is trivial but overnight becomes more significant and who frequently need social services, physical and occupational therapy. The patient who is drunk with a head injury. Every year, a few are sent home too early and found dead in the morning. The list goes on and on, but the point is that Labour's bright idea is going to kill people.

'It's easier to admit patients than to discharge them, and many more patients will now be referred up the line to wait somewhere else in the hospital. But forcing a four-hour turnaround on everyone may just increase inappropriate admissions and create a log-jam on the wards. The main problem blocking up A&E departments is waiting for a bed for those patients who really need it. Little has been done to address this, and the target will only make it worse.'

What a Hunt

11 April 2003

'Some targets are essential. . . . But we set far too many and the beleaguered NHS is suffering under the weight of it all.' So says Lord Hunt of Kings Heath, with the confidence of an ex-junior health minister.

Hunt resigned over the war in Iraq, not in the NHS, but his posthumous reflections recognise that the Government's reforms are destined to fail unless they win over the hearts and minds of the staff. A conference aiming to unite doctors and managers organised by the NHS confederation and the Royal Colleges earlier this month found that many doctors are unhappy and unwilling to implement the Government's 'aggressive and unsophisticated attitude to health reform,' and so make life as hard as possible for middle managers. None of this bodes well for the extra billions being ploughed into the NHS.

As one orthopaedic surgeon put it: 'We are deeply in the mire. Having bust a gut to hit a twelve-month inpatient-wait target by the end of March, we now have a huge backlog of urgent cases who have been disadvantaged.' Another complains that 'the Saturday blitz to clear non-urgent waiting lists has meant old ladies with fractured femurs sitting on the wards.

The more their surgery is delayed, the sicker they get. Mortality in this group has gone up 30%, and those that survive are staying longer, blocking beds for elective cases.' Hunt is right – too many targets are bad for patients. It's a shame he couldn't have been so vociferous in office.

The Limits of Medicine

24 April 2003

The failure of Labour to turn round the NHS and deliver value for our extra billions is not just because of its flawed model of centralist control using simplistic targets, but it's also down to the over-hyping of medicine. Whatever model of healthcare we have, doubling the amount we spend won't make us twice as healthy, because the treatments don't work as well as the pharmaceutical industry would have us believe. As Richard Smith, editor of the *British Medical Journal*, recently observed: 'Medicine is increasingly about complex and multiple interventions in chronically sick patients with marginal improvements.'

Smith's comments were in response to two studies (*BMJ*, January 11). The first looked at trying to stop elderly patients with dementia who had already fallen, from falling again. 274 patients were assessed by doctors, physiotherapists and occupational therapists, and then one group was randomised to receive intervention on every possible risk factor – including balance, drugs, environmental hazards, feet and footwear, and vision. A huge amount of time and effort went into this study and into the active treatment. And yet the result was no improvement compared with conventional care: three-quarters of patients in both groups fell again, and a fifth died.

A more optimistic study from Aberdeen examined the four-year results of a trial of secondary prevention in over 1,300 patients with coronary heart disease. Patients in the intervention group received multiple tests, treatments and advice. The result after four years was 128 deaths and 125 'coronary events' (e.g. heart attacks) in the control group and 100 deaths and 100 events in the intervention group. A modest success story, but not without considerable effort and organisation usually not available outside the constraints of funded research. Getting that level of care in the NHS is near impossible, and so the real-life benefits of much research are far smaller than claimed.

Further evidence of the huge amount of effort required to eke out small benefits is found in research into cervical screening (*BMJ*, April 25). This is the best model of screening we have and saves 1,300 lives a year. But to prevent one death, we have to screen a thousand women for 35 years. And for each life saved, 150 other women have abnormal results, 80 of whom will be referred on for investigations and possible treatment and one woman will die of cervical cancer despite receiving the best-possible screening. Aside from the organisation and workload involved, even good screening creates large amounts of anxiety and treatment for women who are never going to get cancer. And it only stops half of those who are.

For breast screening, the evidence of benefit is far less. In 2001, a prestigious Cochrane review of all the best available studies led the editor of the *Lancet*, Richard Horton, to conclude: 'At present, there is no reliable evidence, from large randomised controlled trials, to support mammography services.' At best, we have to screen a thousand women over 50 for ten years to save one life, and yet many more suffer the anxiety of abnormal results, invasive breast surgery and chemotherapy for no benefit. The popular perception that a pathologist can always make a clear distinction between cancer and non-cancer has always been false. There is a whole spectrum of cell changes that no-one has a clue as to the significance of, but in a litigious society the 'safe' option is to offer aggressive treatment rather than be held up for missing cancer.

Earlier this year, the *Eye* revealed that in 75% of drug trials, anti depressants are no more effective than placebos. Both work, at least in the short term, but sugar tablets are a lot easier to come off. This provoked a large, predominantly supportive response from *Eye* readers. The respected Critical Psychiatry Network is holding a debate in London on June 3 entitled 'Antidepressants are no better than placebos'.[1] With eminent psychiatrists doubting the very few treatments they have, and Labour favouring coercion and control in their mental-health policy, it's a bad time to be mad.

All-Over Massage

8 May 2003

The success of Tony Blair's 'four hours in casualty target' has been helped by advance warning that assessment would take place in the last week of March, allowing managers to divert the required resources for one week only. Figures sent to the *Eye* show that Norfolk and Norwich, Addenbrooke's, Ipswich, West Suffolk and James Paget hospitals all managed to hit the 90% target when the box-tickers were on site, but in the last week in February, none of them did.

The pressure to comply is great, and yet takes no account of the realities of the service. The general manager of A&E at James Paget Hospital (Great Yarmouth) sent a stroppy letter out before target-week admitting that 'extra resources have been obtained' but chastising the staff for the 'extremely disappointing' figures for the previous day. On that day, a senior house officer had to

---

[1] www.critpsynet.freeuk.com/Press2003.htm

repair a very nasty laceration that required debridement and suturing. She did a fantastic job, but it took one and a half hours, taking the patient over the four-hour limit.

A seriously ill intravenous drug addict was also brought in, along with other cases of major trauma, and one senior doctor had to delay treating minor injuries to help. The patient had been on the floor for three days and was critically ill, but had no veins for a drip. It took three-quarters of an hour to cannulate a vein in his foot. The doctors worked their butts off and stayed over their shifts to finish the minor cases. That same week, one doctor came in by mistake when his shift had been changed and stayed (for no pay) because of short-staffing. He also worked the two fourteen-hour shifts over the weekend, seeing 50 patients in one ten-hour spell. His reward? A letter from a manager expressing her extreme disappointment.

One way to reduce waiting times is not to let patients on the list in the first place. Earlier this year Mike Heilbron, a dental surgeon from Muswell Hill, referred a patient to Guy's Hospital for root canal treatment, only to be informed: 'we have temporarily closed the list of referrals until we clear our backlog.' Not to be deterred, Dr Heilbron tried referral to University College London Hospitals NHS Trust: 'The service is particularly oversubscribed and we are not able to offer the patient an appointment.' If you need root canal work in London, you may as well whistle.

Bad Feet

6 June 2003

One consistent feature of the NHS is its pretence of providing a fully comprehensive service whilst quietly jettisoning low-profile 'Cinderella' services. Under the Tories, dentistry and long-term care of the elderly started to fall off the NHS, and

Labour has done little to reverse the trend. The latest non-sexy specialty not to make it to the NHS ball is podiatry, which changed its name from chiropody in a bid to raise its profile. Alas, it hasn't worked.

Badly maintained feet cause a huge amount of discomfort and damage, especially for those too frail to reach them. Without podiatry, they become frailer and even more immobile and unstable, and a vicious circle kicks in. Demand for podiatry in an ageing population is increasing rapidly, with a current caseload of 2.25 million, and the NHS reached maximum capacity in 1995. Faced with the political embarrassment of offering elderly patients nine-month waits for basic foot care, many health authorities have decided not to offer it at all. Services are now restricted to those 'at risk' (largely diabetic), and waiting lists have been quietly culled.

Researcher Mark Russell has unearthed that, in the year 2001–02 more than 550,000 patients were removed from lists, forcing many into the unregulated private sector at £30 a visit. Elderly patients with common foot disorders often require four treatments a year. Many are unable to pay, and a study by Northampton University found that a majority of those denied treatment deteriorate so much that they become 'at risk' within a year.

The Government's response, as ever, is to deny the service has been rationed and that their 'national service frameworks' (NSFs) will insist on proper foot care. Ironically, the new diabetic NSF may actually make things worse. It specifies that all diabetic patients should have access to podiatry services whether they need them or not. So a huge influx of new patients will further swamp the service for annual check-ups with no new money on offer. A nineteen-year-old diabetic with perfect feet can now get free foot care as and when they like, but a 90-year-old with pathological nails and corns who enjoyed free NHS foot care for 30 years now has to go private.

A pragmatic solution would be to be honest about the need to ration healthcare and introduce modest fees for selected NHS services. Mr Russell has calculated that simple foot care could be provided by the NHS with a maximum charge per visit of £5. This part of the service would then become completely self-funding, and far cheaper than going private. Alas, Labour would far rather bury the problem than invite a political row over NHS charges. In a recent *Times* column, health secretary Alan Milburn pledged: 'Reform must deliver not just improved services but a different sort of service – one where users are in the driving seat.' There's not much point being in the driving seat if you can't use the pedals.

JOHN REID
June 2003–May 2005

The alleged response of Dr John Reid on seeing a panicked Tony Blair on reshuffle morning was: 'Oh fuck, not health'. The response of many NHS staff was: 'Oh fuck, not John Reid'. One self-deluded macho reformer gets replaced with another. But despite the bluster, Reid was far more of a glazier than a window-breaker, largely because he wasn't that interested in the detail and hoped his reward for stepping into the health furnace would be a timely move to defence.

Things looked grim at the outset, with the Commission for Health Improvement announcing a record number of 'zero-star' hospitals and negotiations for GP and consultant contracts in stalemate. But Reid proved very adept at pressing the flesh, and amazed everyone by getting both sets of doctors to sign up to new deals. The secret? Offer them lots of money and let someone else figure out how to pay.

Reid was on a spending spree. He may as well have invited Elton John. He paid private companies over the odds to cherry-pick easy NHS operations and, to cap it all, they got paid top-whack whether they fulfilled their contracts or not. Lots more ludicrously expensive Private Finance Initiative contracts were signed off, and a new system of Payment By Results allowed hospitals to hoover up money. Despite the record investment, the English NHS was heading for record debt, but at least Reid realised it. On his departure, he allegedly advised Tessa Jowell: 'Don't go to health. I've spent all the money.' Reid may have had a PhD, but it wasn't in accounting.

PRIVATE EYE
Oh Fuck, Not the Working Time Directive

31 July 2003

One of the most pressing issues for new health secretary, Dr John 'Oh Fuck, Not Health' Reid, is the impending implementation of the European working time directive (EWTD), which could lead to widespread downgrading of local hospitals and completely scupper Labour's NHS Plan.

The EWTD requires that by August 2004, junior doctors should work a maximum of 58 hours a week, with further restrictions on length of shift, rest periods and sleep while on-call, falling to 48 hours by 2009. A survey of 211 hospitals by the Royal College of Physicians has found that 166 'do not have sufficient numbers of specialist registrars to give continuous cover of acute medical admissions'. These hospitals have fewer than ten specialist registrars in medicine, with 44 having fewer than five and, at present, they are completely unable to cope.

The Royal College of Surgeons has also spotted that a drastic reduction in hours in the current system will have a dire effect on training, with many new consultants already unsafe to independently cover all of the operations in their job description. But the biggest challenge may be to anaesthetists. They consume only 3% of hospital resources but contribute to over two-thirds of trust income. One estimate found that to hit the targets in the NHS plan and comply with the EWTD, every graduate from every medical school for the next five years would need to become an anaesthetist.

The Government has a number of options. It could ignore the legislation and run the risk of mass employment law litigation. It could seek to try to delay the legislation, but is unlikely to succeed. It could 'reconfigure' the NHS, by closing or downgrading lots of smaller district general hospitals and ferrying patients into massive hospitals, which would be politically disastrous and renege on a recent pledge to keep the NHS local. Or it could try and parachute large numbers of junior doctors out of large teaching hospitals and into smaller ones, where most end up as consultants anyway.

The latter seems logical, but many junior doctors deliberately choose to avoid acute general medicine in busy district hospitals because the workload is unremitting, the expectations huge, and support and teaching decidedly variable. Hiding in a teaching hospital, doing research and retreating into a very specialised area of medicine is a far more attractive option.

This is the heart of the battle between the Government and doctors. Labour feels that the NHS employs doctors and should therefore dictate precisely where they work and what that work should involve. Doctors want a degree of professional autonomy, to have the power to challenge politically driven targets and want to be free to choose jobs with humane working conditions and good training. It's a stalemate that even John Reid will have difficulty swearing his way out of.

Tooth Fury

15 August 2003
'NHS dentistry seems to be cryogenically frozen on the edge of crisis.' So says an article in the *Health Service Journal*, dating the problems back to the Conservatives' 1991 contract reforms, which caused an exodus of dentists into the private sector. John Major promised everyone access to an NHS dentist, and Tony Blair fell into the same trap at the 1999 Labour party conference. His deadline of September 2001 failed so pitifully that Downing Street backtracked and pretended he just meant everyone could phone up NHS Direct and find out where their nearest NHS dentist is.

The absurdity of this ploy was well publicised last month, with NHS Direct Wales advising dentist-less patients to take a trip to the Mansell Street practice in Carmarthen. One man paid £8.30 to get on the 8.15am bus from Aberaeron, arriving at 9.25am to find himself at the back of a 600-strong queue. Two years on from Tony's pledge, and patients are still having to make hundred-mile round trips to find a dentist or, more likely, stock up on painkillers and do without.

So, where's it all gone wrong? In private medical practice, you get treated more quickly but the standard of care and quality of materials are usually no better than the NHS. In private dentistry, you get speed, better materials and a better standard of care – although you can also get ripped off. Last year, the Audit Commission found that dentistry is 'one of the significant areas of NHS fraud'.

The commission also quoted John Renshaw, British Dental Association executive board chair, as saying: 'The way we work is often driven more by the way we are paid than by the treatment needs of our patients.' The fact that dentists (like doctors) are human, and respond to financial incentives, is unsurprising. The trick is to give them incentives to provide the best possible care on the NHS, a situation which clearly isn't happening.

A report published in UK Dental Care earlier this year found that, for the first time, dentists are receiving more than half of their income from treating private patients. It also found that the number of adults registered for NHS treatment is 1.5 million lower than when Labour took over, and 5 million lower than the Tory peak in 1994. The vast majority of dentists continue with some NHS work and would love to do more, but only if resources are sufficient for them to provide a comparable standard of care to private practice.

The buck for commissioning NHS dentistry, and just about everything else, has now been passed onto beleaguered PCTs, most of whom haven't got a clue how to meet the government criteria on providing 'reasonable dental services'. Adult orthodontic work is near impossible to get on the NHS, and only a public uproar saved the service for children.

As with medicine, the shortage of practitioners has forced the Government's hand. Temporary registration of overseas dentists is being extended, and they can work for eighteen weeks in salaried NHS clinics. Whether these dentists work to the same standards as UK-trained dentists is anybody's guess, because in the scramble to clear the backlog it's unlikely much attention will be paid to the quality of the work.

Education is also urgently needed. Dental hospitals are regularly putting children as young as three under general anaesthetic and removing a dozen rotten milk teeth, and health inequalities in tooth decay are huge. The bottom line with dentistry is that quality costs, and prevention is better than a drill. I've never used a private doctor, but I have a private dentist. And, as he puts it: 'Only floss the teeth you want to keep.'

More Target Tosh

23 August 2003

What do you do if you can't meet the thirteen-week government target for waiting for an appointment? Close the waiting list. This tactic has been adopted by the North West Leeds area adult psychological and therapy service. Those lucky enough to get an initial appointment then have to wait nine to twelve months for treatment because, in the last eight years, the unit has been fully staffed for only two six-month periods. In an understaffed NHS governed by targets, not treatment, the only way to get ticks in all the right boxes is to restrict the service.

The absurdity of the target culture is well articulated by

Richard Harrad, clinical director of Bristol Eye Hospital. He has calculated that 25 patients with diabetes or glaucoma went blind through lack of follow-up, because of the drive to meet new patient appointment targets. Hardly treatment according to clinical need.

As Dr Harrad put it: 'This figure undoubtedly under-estimates the true incidence and of course there is the large backlog of patients still to be seen. One particularly sad case was that of an elderly lady who was completely deaf and relied on signing and lip-reading for communication. She lives with her disabled husband, who, like her, is completely deaf. Her follow-up appointments for glaucoma were delayed several times and during this time her glaucoma deteriorated and she became totally blind.'

In the new NHS, trolleys are re-designated as 'beds on wheels' and corridors and treatment rooms are re-designated as 'pre-admission units' to give the illusion of better care. My nearest four hospitals are bottom of the league table, with not one star between them, but this absurd system takes very little account of clinical performance (which is often excellent in Bristol and Bath).

For most of the NHS targets, there is no evidence that they improve care, but plenty that they distort it. As orthopaedic surgeons at Princess Royal University Hospital, Farnborough put it: 'Why is the same target used for a minor graze as for a major trauma case? We have had numerous examples of patients being admitted purely to avoid breaching the four-hour Accident and Emergency wait. At best this has ended in an immediate discharge for an inappropriate admission with all the attendant increase in costs and decrease in free beds. At worst, the patient is transferred without the resuscitation and immediate treatment they need.'

With such severe financial penalties associated with multiple breaches, the pressure to conform is huge, and it's going to get even worse. By March 1, 2004 all trusts are obliged to admit, transfer or discharge 100% of their casualty patients within four hours. However, a Department of Health memo, dated June 16, suggests a possible opt out: 'Clarification of the definition of 100% is currently being discussed with the professional bodies.'

Dr Phil's Notes

There are supporters of the four-hour casualty wait target, even amongst doctors. It has certainly focused attention on treating patients more quickly, but the key is to allow enough wisdom and flexibility to observe patients for longer if that is the safest thing to do. And don't bother fiddling figures or diverting resources from elsewhere. Managers and NHS staff need to grow up and tell it like it is.

Likewise, Labour deserves some credit for reducing waiting times, but not when it has been at the expense of sicker patients. The test is whether the front line staff agree not just with a target, but how a target is implemented. If they can see the point, it'll be introduced and get results. If they don't, you just get perfunctory care and a tribe of surly robots.

Selling Off the NHS

24 September 2003

So, £2 billion-worth of NHS work is to be handed over to seven private companies (five of them South African or North American) according to health secretary John Reid. He is confident these Independent Sector Treatment Centres (ISTCs) can knock off 250,000 routine operations a lot more quickly than NHS hospitals, and at a price somewhere in between the NHS and UK private hospitals, none of which won significant contracts in the new scheme. Reid claims that consultants are against the scheme because it would reduce their private practice, but the majority of consultants don't do private practice. Their main objections are the effect it will have on NHS hospitals, leaving them as a sink for emergencies, the chronic sick and complex cases too ill to be seen in the private centres.

Reid justifies paying ISTCs substantially more than the NHS because 'the staff will work harder.' This is nonsense, as outlined by one NHS surgeon: 'The stuff they will do in ISTCs is, quite frankly, easy. It only takes twenty minutes or so to see a fit patient with a hernia in clinic, make the diagnosis and discuss the operation. It takes twenty minutes to do the operation and the patient is out of hospital in under four hours. I regard a list of hernia repairs almost as relaxation.

'In contrast, emergencies are frequently extremely ill and require complex investigation, resuscitation and multiple reviews over hours before they are fit enough for surgery, which may also be complex. They are often critically ill afterwards and require intensive input from clinicians. There may be difficult discussions with family about "withdrawing support" and this may take place more than once. ISTC doctors may do more operations but they will be much simpler. And when things go wrong, the patients will come back to us as emergencies.'

ISTCs may well reduce waiting lists for routine operations and make good political headlines, but it seems absurd that they are paid above the going rate to do easier operations. And their contracts are guaranteed, so the companies (and their shareholders) will be paid even if no patients choose to be treated there. If you're going to have competition in the NHS, at least make it fair. And would the money be better spent allowing the NHS to treat them?

New Labour, Old Tory

9 October 2003

'Earlier this year, the Government announced a programme of reform to strengthen and modernise the Health Service. . . . Local hospitals will be able to become self-governing, run by a local board, while remaining completely within the NHS. . . . These hospitals will be locally managed, with much more local pride and commitment, and have much more freedom to take control of their own affairs. At the moment, too many decisions affecting local services are made in Whitehall.'

This Department of Health leaflet sounds almost identical to a Labour press release plugging foundation hospitals. Alas, it dates back to 1990 when the Tories announced the arrival of NHS trusts. The failure of the Tory market reforms to deliver a better service may perhaps explain why health secretary John Reid can't even persuade his own party to back him.

Labour has also adopted the old Tory idea of patient choice. In the nineties, the NHS was divided into purchasers and providers, on the understanding that purchasers could shop around the market on behalf of patients, who would then have free referral in the NHS. In the event, health authorities were obliged to agree block contracts with trusts, which meant most patients had no choice where they went. Getting a health authority to stump up for an extra-contractual referral was near impossible.

Under Labour, the purchaser remains the NHS, but the provider could be anyone you like. In theory, you can choose for your hip to be replaced at an NHS hospital (local or distant), at a private hospital (with an NHS contract), at a diagnostic and treatment centre (private or NHS), or in France. Reid's advantage over the Tories is that he has more money to play with. But choice is only meaningful if you have outcome figures that allow you to fairly compare different hospitals. Until we do, it's pointless.

Anger Management

6 November 2003

A recent BMA survey that found one in three doctors have suffered violent behaviour from patients or relatives of patients in the last year has had some interesting responses. As one casualty registrar put it: 'Is it really only one in three? I've just finished a weekend of nights – physically attacked once, verbally abused six times, mouthfuls of blood spat at myself and nursing colleagues by one charmer, and the first time our team has been threatened by a gang of fifteen bikers who tried to tear down security screens.'

So, what to do about it? The Government's 'zero tolerance' plan (which involves putting up lots of 'zero tolerance' posters) seems to have failed, so the staff are having to take action. As another casualty doctor put it: 'I've been sworn at, punched, kicked, strangled, threatened with a knife, threatened with being shot (over the phone), had a cigarette stubbed out on my arm, been spat at and attacked with a chair. You have several options while confronted by this:

'1. The "Beirut" approach: I spent two months with Glasgow ambulance paramedics as part of my elective. I was in the back of an ambulance with a paramedic travelling down a 40mph road in Coatbridge when the patient grabbed my collar and started shouting at me. The vehicle screeched to a halt, the back doors flew open and the paramedics threw the patient out of the vehicle onto the road. They then told him if he wanted back in he had to behave himself. Shaken, and meek as a lamb, he climbed back in. Glasgow crews refer to Coatbridge as "Beirut" for this reason.

'2. The "only I get to swear in here" approach: "Shut the fuck up or I'll have you arrested and removed." Make sure you have an open escape route in case the patient decides to attack you.

'3. The "retreat and get the fuzz" approach, returning with them as an escort or outside the curtains. Tell the patient that

189

in view of the threat to your safety you will only treat them with the police present.

'4. The "press charges" approach – I got £100 from a punter on top of his £1,000 fine after he took a chair and chased me round an A&E.

'Once you are happy the patient's life is not in immediate danger, refuse to treat them until they behave. Always make an official report, preferably a police one as well. Document why you were unable to treat the patient properly. And as for aggressive or violent relatives – first sign of trouble and I have them all removed (by the police if necessary).'

Private Loss

'If the Government get this right, it could be the death of private practice.' So confided a senior BUPA source over Labour's plans to franchise out substantial amounts of lucrative NHS surgery to independent sector treatment centres. The price per head is significantly more than the NHS, but significantly less than the usual private fee. So why pay to go private when you can do it on the NHS for free? While this approach will doubtless reduce waiting lists for hips, hernias and cataracts, and make nice profits for private shareholders, the NHS can't compete because it can't cherry-pick and turn away the critically ill, uncontrollably angry, chronically sick and anyone with MRSA. Maybe we should ferry round busloads of wandering, MRSA-carrying octogenarians and pissed bikers to private treatment centres, to level the playing field.

Informed Choice?

20 November, 2003
'For patients, choice matters, and we must make existing choices

real and look to extend these.' So says health secretary John Reid. Labour's vision of a consumerist NHS is for patients to book on-line for a GP appointment and choose their hospital treatment from a large selection of providers (private, NHS and foreign) based on 'access and outcome information measures'. Fine sentiments, but will they work in the real world?

An early pioneer of patient consumerism was a GP who left a trough full of antibiotics in his waiting room with a 'help yourself' sticker above it. Rather than being hailed as a trailblazer, he was censured by the GMC. As one Essex GP puts it: 'all this guff about patient choice leaves out the crucial word "informed". The reason patients consult us in the first place is because we are better informed than they are. That's why I have a prescription pad and they don't.'

Alas, this rather defensive view doesn't work either. It costs £300,000 to train a doctor, and each dishes out over £3 million worth of treatment in a career. Yet at best only half of patients take sufficient medication for it to be effective. It's a phenomenal waste of time and money, and the Government could save a fortune by launching an 'if you don't want the tablets, don't bother the doctor' campaign.

Instead, the DoH is ignoring patients with medical conditions and focusing choice on surgery. Patients will be given information such as average wait for an appointment, average wait for surgery, 30-day mortality and morbidity rates, number of stars, latest hospital inspection report and position in the Dr Foster Opal Fruit Beezer Homes League Table – and then asked to choose. Those who still wish to go to the hospital with the easiest car parking will be allowed to, but Labour hopes enough patients will shop around to introduce a market discipline into the NHS.

The Tories tried this and it bombed because there was neither enough money nor capacity in the system. Labour is trying to force it through with more money but still very little capacity. As Dr Richard Lawson, a GP in Somerset, puts it: 'Ten days ago, I helped a patient exercise her right of choice regarding hospitals. It took over two hours and involved about twenty phone calls. . . . We can only extend choice if there are adequate resources, and there are more urgent things to buy first, like basic mental health services or outpatient appointments that are not postponed ten times.'

Another key stumbling block is IT – the technology for e-booking and an 'electronic spine' that allows access to NHS records anywhere in the service may one day arrive, but there will always be worries about confidentiality (what price a tabloid bribing a maintenance engineer to gain access to celebrity records?). A more pressing concern is that there are no standards or syllabus for medical record-keeping. Many are in a shockingly illegible state, and different words mean different things to different professions – without uniformity of record-keeping, the information entered on the spine could be dangerously misleading, yet no-one has addressed this.

The Government, alas, continues to plough money into consumerism with little proof of value. Patient Advocacy and Liaison Services have no real power to stand up to the trusts that employ them. The latest vogue is to 'understand the patient experience'. So we now have a 'Commission for Patient and Public Involvement in Health' who'll shortly be seeding the NHS with 'involvement forums' to 'democratise the grass roots of health.'

As one doctor observed: 'Before my endoscopy list last week, I was asked to see a man from the Cancer Network. He was pleasant and polite, but seemed a bit clueless. He was a "Cancer Network Facilitator" who was "tracking the journey" of patients with cancer. He was apparently responsible to a "Cancer Network Facilitator Co-ordinator". When I enquired what he was doing, he thought for a minute and then suggested he had to measure something.

'He thought that having only just started, he would need six months or so in post to enable him to "focus" on a project which would help cancer patients. He has no previous medical experience, and is apparently employed by the PCT. He is paid more than the sister who runs the unit. One despairs . . .'

Second Thoughts

2 January 2004

On April 28, 1997, 60 esteemed doctors signed a letter to the *Daily Mirror*, advising readers on how to vote to save the NHS: 'As doctors, we see mounting evidence each day that the NHS is no longer able to care for the nation's sick. Waiting lists grow, bureaucracy has snowballed, the sick lie on trolleys. Doctors and nurses are in despair. Accounting comes before care. . . . Your treatment depends not on your needs but upon where you live. . . . The internal market is a cancer eating away at your National Health Service. Left untreated it will destroy that service . . . if the Tories get in again, the NHS as we know it will disappear. To protect its future we urge you to vote Labour.'

Tony Blair was so chuffed with this endorsement that he sent Professor Vincent Marks, then chairman of the BMA, a thank-you letter and invited him to sit with him at a press conference. Blair also came up with his risible election-eve claim that 'there are just 24 hours to save the NHS'. Nearly seven years later, he's still trying and with policies the Tories wouldn't have dared to introduce. In opposition, Labour ridiculed PFI financing but were swiftly converted to it in office. Despite ex-health secretary Alan Milburn's pledge that 'the NHS is not for sale', all new hospital building projects are farmed out to private companies. This has undoubtedly resulted in lots of new hospitals, and richer architects, but nearly all are too small, the risk transfer is inadequate and the loan repayments so high that lower-profile areas of the NHS will suffer for years to come.

Even more contentious is that £2 billion-worth of lucrative NHS elective surgery is to be offered to private treatment centres largely owned by overseas companies. According to Labour philosophy, these private companies will not be competing with the NHS, they will be part of it, and care will be driven not by the hated internal market, but by patient choice. By negotiating a single tariff for an operation, wherever it is performed, Labour argue that the NHS will not be driven by a market based on cost, but purely on consumer choice. This seems unlikely. The cost of an operation may be fixed, but patients vary enormously in their fitness for surgery and some hospitals or treatment centres may decide to cherry-pick the easier cases and then charge a price that is less than the tariff. And there will always need to be a financially disadvantaged NHS safety net to take on the difficult cases and pick up the pieces when the private sector screws up. Also, private companies will want a guaranteed workload before setting up treatment centres, and it is hard to see how such a block contract equates with patient choice.

It is also hard to see the distinction between the Tory vision of 'self-governing trusts' and Labour's foundation hospitals which, despite their neutered powers, will still have unfair financial advantages compared to their neighbours. As with the Tory internal market, the playing field is not level. Hospitals in deprived areas with more complex caseloads find it harder to hit the 'three star' foundation target than those in more privileged areas. Others get a helping hand. As the *Health Service Journal* revealed (December 18, 2003), Alan Milburn intervened in the proposed star rating of South Durham Healthcare Trust because 'it serves the Prime Minister's constituency.' And his own. By some mysterious recalculation, it was upgraded from two to three stars, making it eligible for a £1 million capital-funding grant and giving it significant freedom from government control.

Many of the 60 doctors who endorsed Labour seven years ago are having second thoughts. Professor Marks contacted 52 of them and has written to the *Eye* with the results: 'In my view, the decision to create foundation hospitals and (private) treatment centres is more detrimental to the future of the NHS than any other act since it was first created. The fact that over 90% of former strong Labour supporters with genuine knowledge of the situation feel the same should give Blair cause for thought.' But of course it won't. Happy New Year.

Bribing Doctors

30 January 2004

The quality and outcomes framework at the heart of the new GP contract should be a good thing, concentrating on managing chronic diseases better and preventing strokes, heart disease and cancer. But instead of relying on doctors' professionalism to treat patients as best they can, Labour is 'incentivising' them with money. Once you start bribing doctors to behave in a certain way, medicine becomes coercive and the neutrality of professional doctors is undermined. What works for double-glazing doesn't work for diabetes.

As one GP put it: 'Yesterday I went to a meeting about preparing for the new contract. A couple of respected local colleagues gave a presentation on how to earn the most out of it. They explained how they chased up patients via their repeat prescriptions, how their receptionists quizzed people about their smoking habits, and they provided estimates of what they might earn if they hit all their targets. The room was full of intelligent, hard-working, earnest men and women, eager to do their utmost for their patients. But at best they were acting like a bunch of sales reps at a conference, learning how to get out there and flog the product, lapping up all the little tricks of the trade that previously no-one knew of. At worst they were a bunch of performing seals, expected to jump through hoops and balance beach balls in the hope of someone chucking them a sprat as reward.

'What has my profession come to? No consultant would stoop this low, to sit and listen to someone tell him his income depended on making his patients sign an "informed dissent" form if they didn't want to take another blood pressure pill. A pox on the General Practitioners' Committee for a contract that reduces us to a bunch of snake-oil salesmen. A pox on all the "yes" voters for agreeing to it. I am thoroughly embarrassed to be part of this.'

Cheap Choice

26 February 2004

The Government's emphasis on increasing patient choice sounds like a vote-winner but will it make the NHS any safer? As GP Dr Nick Summerton warns: 'Choice is not necessarily synonymous with a better-quality service. Patients may choose to have their warfarin treatment monitored in the community, have their skin lesion excised in general practice or have sigmoidoscopy performed in the PCT diagnostic unit. But if the warfarin monitoring service has not signed up to the external quality control scheme, the skin lesion is not submitted for pathological examination or the sigmoidoscope used is rigid rather than flexible, then patients are being short-changed. Sadly these are all real examples. . . . An ineffective or unsafe service is not a choice I want to offer to my patients.'

Ex-health minister and now chair of the National Patient Safety Agency (NPSA) Lord Hunt has similar concerns:

'Patients should consider their safety when exercising their right to choice of treatment. Or would they prefer to assume – as they do in the airline industry – that safety is a given and choice can be made on the basis of other factors?' Alas, the NHS is a far more complex and under staffed organisation than the airline industry and safety can never be a given. Each year, 10% of patients are injured by the NHS, and the equivalent of a jumbo jetload of patients die each week from preventable errors in hospitals alone. Maybe if NHS staff died with our patients, we'd take a bit more care.

Heart surgery is the one example where the NHS is getting its act together in providing meaningful information to patients. It took the Bristol disaster to kick-start it and even then, there is has been huge difficulty in attracting sufficient money for audit. Some centres have managed to translate complex statistics into information that patients can actually use (e.g. Papworth Hospital's newsletters and website http://www.papworth-hospital.org.uk/). Elsewhere it is almost impossible to find accurate, user-friendly information on the safety and quality of NHS services. Without it, the entire patient choice programme could be a huge and very costly stab in the dark.

Secret Drug Trials and HRT

20 April 2004

In 1977 Sir Richard Doll, the epidemiologist who has saved millions of lives by proving that smoking causes lung cancer and heart disease, co-wrote an editorial in the *British Medical Journal* demanding that the results of all clinical trials should be made public, and not just those which the pharmaceutical industry wishes us to see. As a pioneer of the randomised controlled trial (RCT), he recognised the dangers of selection bias and the importance of assessing all the evidence when considering the risks and benefits of new drugs. So why, nearly 30 years later, are companies still allowed to keep the effects of licensed drugs a secret?

The damage that such secrecy does is well documented. Back in 1980, the Finnish researcher Elina Hemminki showed that among studies submitted for new drug licences, those that found side-effects were less likely to be published. For over a decade, heart attack patients were given drugs to prevent heart rhythm disturbance, until in 1990 it was discovered they were killing more Americans each year than died in Vietnam. If the evidence had not been buried from the start, the tragedy could well have been avoided.

Recently, the *Eye* highlighted that anti-depressant medication is less powerful, and has more side-effects, than the selective release of trial information by the drug industry would have us believe. There is now clear evidence from the Swedish Medical Products Agency of this biased reporting favouring new drugs. Without compulsory publication of all trials from the outset, we often have to wait decades for the truth, from the slow and haphazard reporting of adverse events.

The most recent 'scare' into the safety of Hormone Replacement Therapy (HRT) is a case in point. The potential HRT market is vast, with women living on average 30 years after the menopause. HRT has been used since the 1950s, but it took nearly 30 years to spot the increased risk of womb cancer from oestrogen-only drugs. Progestogen was added in the 1980s, and these combined preparations have been amongst the most heavily marketed in history. A flawed, but at the time convincing, observational study of 120,000 nurses provided evidence that HRT was not only good for relieving menopausal symptoms (it is) but it also might protect against heart disease.[1]

---

[1] Nurses' Health Study. Postmenopausal hormone therapy and mortality. *N Engl J Med* 1997; 336: 1769–75.

This important benefit was thought to far outweigh the possible slight increase in the risk of breast cancer.

Every other page in the medical press contained an absurd advert for HRT. Campaign symbols included a hair dryer (Kliofem), a chained suffragette (Evorel), a dancing saxophonist (Premique) and, most unwisely, a gaping pink oyster (Estring). Nearly all post-menopausal women were encouraged to give HRT a try. Five years ago, I spoke (and lost) at a drug-sponsored debate to oppose the mass medicalisation of the menopause. Opposing me was Professor David Purdie, a consultant gynaecologist, who spoke of HRT as a great achievement: 'There are oestrogen receptors all over the body, and HRT in those who need it has benefits for bone, heart, arteries, mental and nervous function which greatly outweigh the increased risks.'

Supporting me was Dr Ellen Grant, who observed that 'the time course of the breast cancer epidemic in developed countries correlates uncomfortably well with the changes in sex hormone prescribing.' Alas, it took until 2002 to prove it, when a large randomised controlled trial – the only safe way to assess new drugs – found evidence that combined HRT increases the risk of breast cancer, coronary heart disease, stroke and venous clots.[2] A subsequent huge study in the *Lancet* last year found that combined HRT may double the risk of breast cancer with long-term use, and of heart disease in the first year of use.[3]

The drug industry is now desperately ferreting around for evidence from smaller trials to demonstrate that select sub-groups of women may be safe on HRT, but this misses the point

[2] Writing Group of the Women's Health Initiative. Risks and benefits of estrogen plus progestin in healthy postmenopausal women. *JAMA* 2002; 288: 942–5.

[3] Million Women Study Collaborators. Breast cancer and hormone-replacement therapy in the million women study. *Lancet* 2003; 362: 419–27.

entirely. The evidence of the risks of HRT has been around for years, but well hidden. Hemminki and Oxford epidemiologist Klim McPherson, distrustful of the biases in observational studies, meticulously analysed all the available randomised controlled trials on HRT and published their results in 1997.[4] They found that HRT did not protect against heart disease, and if anything increased the risk. The findings were ridiculed by HRT experts, and dismissed as being selective as they didn't have access to all the studies.

So they tried to gain access to the unpublished data but only managed to in Finland, via the High Court. In the UK, they were not able to access the secret trial data of drug companies, even though it affects the health of millions of women. However, the six unpublished Finnish trials showed that the relative increased risk of heart disease on combined HRT was 1.78, which matches well with the results of the large RCT finally published five years later.

In America the conservative estimate is that each year, combined HRT is responsible for 1,400 cases of breast cancer, 1,200 cases of heart disease, and 1,400 cases of stroke—against 860 fewer hip fractures and 1,000 fewer cases of colorectal cancer. There is no doubt it relieves symptoms of the menopause, which in some women can be very distressing, but it is equally true that millions of women have made misinformed choices for several decades. And no-one ever died of a hot flush. The lessons are simple and unchanged since Doll first advocated them: randomised controlled trials are the best way to assess the risks and benefits of drugs, but only if all of them are made public.

[4] Hemminki E, McPherson K. Impact of postmenopausal hormone therapy on cardiovascular events and cancer: pooled data from clinical trials. *BMJ* 1997; 315: 149–53.

Payment by Results?

20 May 2004

Shortly after health secretary John Reid took up the post, he was accosted by civil servants desperate to explain how 'payment by results' (PBR) would revolutionise the NHS. An hour later, he admitted he 'didn't understand a word'. A year later, Reid may well know what it means but, as with the rest of his health reforms, he has no idea if it'll work. Superficially, PBR sounds simple enough – you pay providers of healthcare a fixed price for any given treatment. Those who traditionally charge more than this tariff have to cut their costs, those who charge less make a profit.

Hospitals still have to compete for the business of the PCTs, but on the basis of quality rather than cost. In theory, a hospital that provides better-quality care (e.g. demonstrable safety record, clean wards) and can throw in a few extras (e.g. free transport) should take business away from its neighbour, which may then go bust (unless it happens to be in a Labour constituency in election year, in which case it will be bailed out by the Treasury). PBR has the potential to drive up quality, increase activity and keep costs down, but there are a number of reasons why it could all go pear-shaped . . .

Too Much Too Soon . . .

The time frame is absurdly ambitious. By 2008, the vast majority of a hospital's income will supposedly depend on PBR, covering all accident and emergency cases, critical care, inpatient and outpatient care. In America, where PBR runs on a less grand scale, the largest hospital department is dedicated to income generation and coding. To ensure correct payment, every case has to be correctly coded by breaking it up into a number of 'healthcare resource groups' (HRGs), to ensure that even the most complex treatment is adequately rewarded.

This in itself is a complex business. For example, the HRG for coronary bypass amalgamates 52 types of procedure and the potential for coding error is huge. Yet the NHS is already well known for gross inaccuracies in its data collection; when the audit commission did spot-checks on data quality in 55 trusts last year, seventeen got the lowest (one star) rating. PBR is also critically dependent on the support of clinical staff and the success of the equally error-prone NHS IT programme.

Purchasers too may have difficulty making PBR work. PCTs control most of the NHS budget and are supposed to strike a hard bargain on behalf of patients. But a recent survey found that only a third of them have dedicated finance directors and only one has a full-time IT director. Unsurprisingly, PCTs have been unable to stand up to the bullying tactics of the new foundation trusts, who have tied them into long-term contracts before PBR has been properly assessed.

Playing the System . . .

Foundation trusts have to succeed, so Labour has given them unfair advantages. By being able to borrow against capital, they can kick-start new building more quickly than other hospitals. And by switching to PBR a year earlier than their competitors, they gain windfall profits to plough back into even better facilities to stuff their neighbours. And if they still screw up, the DoH has set aside a £40 million 'risk pool' to prevent bankruptcy of the chosen ones.

Care Out of the Community . . .

The American 'Kaiser' model of healthcare that Tony Blair salivates over invests heavily in community services, prevention and ensuring patients only get admitted to hospital as a very last resort. But under PBR, there will be a tendency for cash-strapped hospitals to see and admit patients more often than necessary because – just like hugely expensive private medicine – each 'episode of care' will attract a fee.

The onus will be on PCTs to query the bills and develop more community services to prevent costly admissions, but at present they're just not up to the task. As it stands, payment by results just means payment by activity, with no check on whether the treatment is necessary. According to the National Audit Office, last year 71 trusts did not achieve 'financial stability' and 51 had 'significant debts'. With so many hospitals struggling to survive, PBR could be just as competitive, divisive and costly as the Tory internal market.

No Cutting Time

17 June 2004

Would you want to be operated on by a newly qualified consultant surgeon? In a recent poll of the existing crop of senior surgeons, those most in a position to know, an alarming two-thirds said they wouldn't.[1] And further down the tree, the skill levels of junior surgeons have been described as 'very shallow'.[2] The reasoning seems simple enough. In the old days, surgeons worked over 30,000 hours between senior house officer and consultant, gaining a huge amount of experience. Now, it's down to 8,000 hours and will, when the European working time directive comes into full force, fall to 6,000.[3] So new surgeons just don't get the cutting time to pass muster.

[1] Training in the Calman era: What consultants say *Bull R Coll Surg Eng* 2002; 84(10): 345–7.
[2] An Audit of the Operative Skills of SHOs on BST programmes. *Ann R Coll Surg Eng* 2001; 83(suppl.): S326–7.
[3] No Time to Train Surgeons. *British Medical Journal* 2004; 328: 418–19.

Alas, the 'I worked 120 hours a week and it never did me any harm' argument doesn't stand up either. Medicine, and surgery in particular, is littered with the victims of self-imposed workaholism (hence the high percentage of depressed, divorced alcoholics). And as surviving consultant surgeon David Reilly puts it: 'There was no golden age of surgical training. There was certainly more time as a junior doctor; time to mature, or time to rot. And it was apparent that there were some staggeringly bad surgeons appointed under the old system, as well as some highly experienced and motivated ones.'

Also, much of the 120-hour week of old was spent doing meaningless repetitive tasks, propping up the NHS and flying by the seat of your pants, rather than receiving high-quality instruction from your consultant, who often wasn't even in the hospital. However, if we're going to produce competent surgeons in a much shorter time frame, it's clear that a lot of emphasis and resource has to be given to improving the training, and in a ratings-obsessed NHS desperate to cut waiting lists in time for the next election, this just isn't happening.

The largest ever survey of senior house officers in orthopaedic surgery found that a third were not taught at all in theatre or clinic.[4] This is all the more alarming when, by 2010, the NHS is facing a projected 63% increase in knee replacements and a 22% increase in hip replacements. Labour's short-term solution is to farm these operations out to treatment centres, private hospitals and overseas, where there is no obligation to train NHS surgeons. So instead of growing our own talent, we may become utterly dependent on the private sector and abroad.

Trainees often take longer to perform operations, and if a dedicated consultant is supervising them, he or she can't be operating elsewhere. But when the pressure to reduce lists is so

[4] Education and Training for SHOs. British Orthopaedic Association 2002.

great, training just doesn't happen. Consultants are also worried that they carry the can (i.e. position in the published league table) for their trainees' results, and so many are reluctant to let trainees take on anything but the simplest cases.

Even the Royal College of Surgeons has been forced to speak out. As president Sir Peter Morris puts it: 'We have been pressing for dedicated training lists and clinics, regretfully without much success. To deliver training and ensure patient safety with the current staff shortages, existing trainers must be adequately supported with time to teach and train. This will inevitably impact on service throughput.'

Alas, throughput trumps training in Labour's NHS and it's the most junior doctors who suffer. As ex-junior leader Paul Thorpe puts it: 'There is a near total disregard by hospitals of the training needs of SHOs.' The Government can argue that there is no hard evidence that the current crop of new surgeons are any worse than in previous years, but alas in surgery there is very little hard evidence of anything. Despite the fall-out from the Bristol disaster and a clutch of incompetent gynaecologists, not nearly enough resource has gone into improving quality and safety. Instead, Blair is obsessed with treating as many people as possible and offering patients choice to take up spare capacity. But if the choice is between three inexperienced surgeons who don't know what they're doing, is it really worth having?

How to Die

26 July 2004
The verdict of the House of Commons' health committee that 300,000 people each year are denied 'a good death' is old news to the Voluntary Euthanasia Society. The Scottish wing, EXIT, has for some time been running workshops on 'self-deliverance', which include 'the latest how-to methods for dying safely'.

A common misconception for those who wish to end it all is that a single pill will do it quickly and humanely. The human body is generally quite resilient to death. Harold Shipman, whose actions have done incalculable harm to palliative care and the voluntary euthanasia movement, had to use large doses of injected opiates. Similarly, Swiss clinics run by organisations such as Dignitas use large doses of barbiturates.

For those unwilling or unable to fly to Switzerland, EXIT workshops favour a dignified DIY death through slow asphyxiation (cutting off oxygen from the brain). Methods advocated in their July newsletter ('no substitute for attending a workshop') include the use of a ratchet ('available from hardware shops and superstores such as B&Q') to compress the carotid arteries rather than the windpipe ('painful') or just the jugular veins (which leaves your face 'congested and purple').

The ratchet has a 'quick release' tie down which is 'useful for practice runs' but 'make sure you know how to work it properly! Death normally occurs very soon (within minutes) of applying the tie down.' The ratchet method is also 'not for the faint of heart who may be considering, at the back of their mind, a cry for help'.

Another method is to put on a painter's mask and immerse yourself in a very large plastic bag (preferably down to the knees) secured by rubber bands around the neck. The mask stops the bag from obstructing breathing, and so you achieve a gentler unconsciousness. You can also use a pair of tights and a wooden spoon to deliver yourself. You turn the spoon to tighten the neck ligature of the tights: 'Bending forward increases the diameter of the neck and thus the constrictive effect of the tights ... the method can be achieved relatively unobtrusively – some small convulsions are likely between passing out and death, but it might pass easily unnoticed.'

That there is a need for these workshops at all is a sad reflection on our treatment of the irreversibly and terminally sick. Very few people wish to be seen shitting and pissing the bed in front of the family when their mind's gone to putty, and yet thousands suffer degrading and prolonged deaths each year. And those who engage in mercy killings, such as 100-year-old Bernard Heginbotham, still get hauled through the courts.

For all Labour's guff about extending patient choice, the one area where it truly matters – when, where and how you die – is still a huge political taboo that is pushed to the back of the queue. 55% of deaths still occur in hospital, when most people express the wish to be at home, and palliative care provision is alarmingly unequal. For example, North Yorkshire gets 20,500 hours of Marie Curie nursing a year but West Yorkshire – four times the size – gets only 11,000. And after Shipman, we'll need to double the non-existent nurses to go through all the drug-safety checks. No wonder people are reaching for the ratchet.

Returning to Practice

24 August 2004

My recent return to general practice seems an apt time to reflect on the state of the National Health Service. It isn't national, it's not a coherent service and it's got very little to do with health. Patients still come in with ear wax and self-limiting illness, and about half of them are overweight. Some of those that need referral onwards are sent to privately owned treatment centres, often without their GP's knowledge. Even though it's our duty to make sure patients get a good service, we're given no information as to the safety and quality of the treatment. But at least it's quicker.

Like the rest of the NHS, general practice itself is being carved up into hundreds of individual tasks which can then be individually coded and costed as a prelude to privatisation. In theory, GPs can then choose whether they wish to do a task for the price offered (e.g. monitor patients on blood-thinning drugs) but in order to claim the fee, they have to stick to strict protocols and keep meticulous, repetitive records. If they choose to opt out, their local PCT is obliged to open the market to other providers, often private, who think they can do the job at that price. The results are predictable; companies will cherry-pick easy cases but complicated ones will get bounced back to the GP.

GPs could refuse, but in practice it's hard to turn down a distressed and confused elderly patient with multiple illnesses and tablets who is in danger of having a major bleed if she gets the dose of warfarin wrong. In a sense, GPs have for decades been their own worst enemies by providing an extensive, holistic but largely unmonitored service much more cheaply than any private company could do. And although a majority of GPs signed up to their new contract, many did so for the chance of opting out of 24-hour responsibility for their patients, rather than a desire to anally document and claim for each of the vast range of tasks they've been doing anyway since the inception of the NHS.

Labour's NHS has become entirely preoccupied with treating diseases, modifying risks and counting all there is to count, rather than focusing on the outcomes that matter. Many patients benefit from simply having someone who listens and accepts them as they are. Most GPs hate being judgemental and forcing medicalisation on people who don't want it, because study after study shows it doesn't work (for example, only a third of patients on long-term medication take it properly). Patients want more face-to-face time with GPs, but they're getting less, and consultations are now interrupted with 'We'd better just pop you on the scales' and 'Do you mind if I just check your blood pressure?' It then takes another five minutes putting all these numbers into the appropriate computer template to claim the fee for measuring them.

GPs now see fewer patients than they used to and fill the time with administrative and management tasks to justify their value to the Government. But the true value of what they do has always been rooted in empathy and support and all the other fluffy things that we can't easily measure. All the extra investment in the NHS is giving us a lot more numbers to count and regale us with come election time, but I doubt the patients are getting much healthier and the GPs are grumpy as hell at being forced to administer a style of doctoring they don't believe will work. Apart from that, it's great to be back.

The Hyde Six

8 September 2004

Not every GP who signed off Harold Shipman's cremation forms has been reported to the GMC. Those who were deemed by the inquiry to have done the job adequately (i.e. spoke to Shipman after the death, examined the body properly and contacted the relatives) have been excused, but they still weren't able to spot the work of a serial killer. So, little will be gained from demonising six neighbouring GPs who didn't spot what Shipman was up to either.

Like every doctor I know, I've never made a meticulous examination of a corpse when I've filled in cremation forms. We could reasonably be expected to spot a machete in the back but not to go over the body with a fine-tooth comb to spot puncture points which in the vast majority of cases will have been from therapeutic drug injections. When doctors phoned Shipman, he didn't admit to murdering his patients with massive opiate injections. And at the time, phoning the relatives to corroborate the GP's story was neither obligatory nor common practice. The profession, for good or bad, ran on the mutual trust of colleagues.

Getting the cause of death wrong is surprisingly common. Post-mortem (PM) examinations find that doctors get it wrong between 30 and 50% of the time. We often write 'broncho-pneumonia' or 'ischaemic heart disease' on the death certificate but it owes as much to informed guesswork as anything else. Alas, the over-reaction to the widespread practice of organ retention has made it even less likely for relatives to consent to PMs. Many people die without us ever knowing the true cause of death.

So, aside from the sheer volume of Shipman's deaths, which one of the GPs reported to the coroner and police (who found nothing amiss), could they reasonably be expected to suspect he was a murderer? The routine rubber-stamping of cremation forms was such a widespread practice at the time that dozens of other GPs are now threatening to bring the GMC to a standstill by reporting themselves for being equally negligent. And any GPs sitting on the Professional Conduct Committee will surely be thinking: 'There but for the grace of God...'

Some GPs are refusing to countersign cremation forms now, either in protest or because they deem that £50 'ash cash' for driving to the funeral parlour, examining the body, phoning the GP and now phoning the distressed relatives to invite their suspicions isn't worth the risk of censure should they fail to spot a well-disguised murder. It also seems likely that many more GPs will refer cases to the understaffed coroner, even if they fall outside the official referral guidelines, to cover their backs.

Two of the GPs reported to the GMC have retired from practice post-Shipman, one with anxiety and depression. Others have been working their butts off in Hyde trying to re-establish the trust that Shipman destroyed. Dragging them to the GMC when most other GPs at that time would have behaved likewise is unlikely to achieve anything constructive, and may further deprive the patients of GPs in an area where recruitment is hardly booming.

The Last of the Single-Handers

21 September 2004

Under Labour's health reforms, most power rests with PCTs, which control 75% of the NHS budget. The initial pretence was for GPs themselves to become the key decision-makers, but their role in the PCTs was swiftly marginalised by career NHS managers who are forced to implement the Government's mantra of patient choice and a 'mixed market economy'. This thin disguise for privatisation is now so transparent that PCTs have been ordered by the Department of Health to offer at least 'one independent option' to NHS patients undergoing routine surgery by December 2005.

Patients haven't asked for this, and indeed most would prefer to go to their local NHS hospital if only it had the capacity and the parking. And when patients do choose a service the PCT isn't interested in, they have to fight to save it. The Government has long had it in for single-handed GPs, with Tony Blair announcing to the Commons on July 3, 2002: 'There has been a move over time away from single-handed practices so as to improve the quality of care that people receive. That has been based on a great deal of evidence over a long time.'

This is complete bollocks; no such evidence exists and indeed smaller practices score highly on many of the quality targets in the new GP contract, particularly patient satisfaction and disease management. But PCTs have taken it upon themselves to close such practices because they don't fit in with the Labour model of primary care: a huge group practice with ten GPs, three dentists (all private) and a McDonald's.

Sorry to Keep Going on About This

4 November 2004

It's now nearly thirteen years since the *Eye* suggested all cardiac surgeons should publish their figures. The Kennedy inquiry agreed, provided they were 'robust, rigorous and risk adjusted' to ensure surgeons aren't penalised for taking on more difficult patients. And the Government and the Society of Cardiothoracic Surgeons (SCTS) promised, in July 2001, that this information would be in the public domain for individual surgeons by April 2004. So where is it?

Health minister John Hutton was itching to get his hands on the statistics, doubtless so he could stick it in a league table and brand surgeons with another absurdly simplistic Labour star rating. He blames the SCTS for not delivering, but doing audit properly is both expensive and unsexy. Trust managers divert even ring-fenced money elsewhere, with the result that Professor Sir Bruce Keogh, president-elect of the SCTS, had to type out the most recent 352-page mortality report single-handedly while on annual leave: 'I have had no support of any kind from anyone apart from one small commercial company.'

Cardiac surgeons have an unbelievably stressful job without having all this dumped on them. As one put it: 'You've got to be operating at peak performance when you're inside someone's chest. If Michael Schumacher had to collect all the performance data for his Ferrari, analyse it and type it up single-handedly the night before a race, he'd be a shit driver.' Keogh has only raw data to go on – many of the NHS's 220 adult cardiac surgeons still don't have the facilities and expertise to adjust it for risk – but the good news is that none of them appear to be dangerously below average on his analysis. But until more accurate figures are collected, individuals will not be named.

The DoH has finally made this cardiac surgery data collection compulsory for trusts, but it needs to extend it to all specialties if its 'choice agenda' is going to be anything other than meaningless. To offer patients a choice of five different surgical teams by December 2005 without having any accurate comparative data on how to choose between them is pointless. Doctors too want this information; if we don't know how we are performing, how can we ever improve? But the real test for MPs and the media is whether it can process the complexities of this information without resorting to bullying and snap public judgement.

The omens are not good. The All-Party Parliamentary Group on Cancer recently concluded that GPs don't refer patients quickly enough and that we should go on 'cancer education programmes'. This was widely reported in the media as 'GPs are crap at spotting cancer.' When doctors miss the obvious (e.g. fail to refer a man who's peeing blood), it's indefensible, but cancer is often far harder to spot at an early stage in a six-minute consultation for an 80-year-old woman with diabetes, depression and irritable bowel who's feeling a bit off-colour. On average, in only four in every 10,000 of our consultations do patients have cancer.

A far more common scenario is for patients with suspected cancer to be referred to hospital to be seen within the two-week target, only to wait months for their subsequent investigations (colonoscopy, barium enema etc.) because the target was introduced without the extra resources to cope with the demand. Some die waiting, others live because they phone the hospital, make a fuss and insist they're seen earlier. In the NHS, it's survival of the loudest.

One Step Forward . . .

18 March 2005
Well done to the 25 heart surgeons in north-west England who have published three years of data on coronary artery bypass

graft and aortic valve replacement in the *British Medical Journal* (March 5). The figures are adjusted for risk so as not to discriminate against those who take on harder surgery in sicker patients. And all of the results compared well with the national average.

Contrast this spirit of openness and proven competence from heart surgeons with the audit of endocrine surgeons carried out by the Royal College of Surgeons on behalf of the British Association of Endocrine Surgeons (BAES). Contributing to this audit is an obligation of membership of BAES and information on three procedures – surgical removal of the thyroid, parathyroid and adrenal glands – is collected. So far, so good. But alas, this is done on anonymised returns. Surgeons are allocated a number and when the audit is published only the individual surgeon can identify him or herself and decide whether any action is appropriate.

The absurdity of this is apparent when the results of the 2000–02 audit are analysed. This has thus far only been circulated to BAES members, but I've seen the results for thyroid and parathyroid surgery and there are an alarming number of unidentifiable surgeons dabbling with this highly complex neck surgery. Some are averaging one (or fewer) operations a year. When I asked a BAES executive committee member if he would allow such a surgeon to operate on him, or a member of his family, the answer was an obvious 'no'. And yet he seemed powerless to do anything about it.

A start would be to kick the dabblers out of BAES. The National Institute of Clinical Excellence has recently published guidelines for the head and neck cancer services, stressing the need for a specialist approach, and BAES has its own guidelines for thyroid surgery which stipulates that 'all thyroid surgery should be performed by surgeons with a special interest and training in thyroid surgery and whose volume of work is sufficient to maintain their relevant skills.' And yet BAES has members who clearly flout this advice.

The climate in which surgeons now operate is tough – while physicians and GPs regularly get away with mixing up the blue pill with the purple pill, surgical errors are much harder to hide. Reductions in junior doctors' hours have meant that surgeons are far less experienced than before, and new consultants don't have the competence to take on the full range of operations expected of them. 50% of surgeons currently suspended are those within six months of taking up their consultant posts, and although the process of investigation is supposed to be 'blame neutral', many careers are being ended before they begin.

The tragedy is that in many cases, surgeons are competent across a range of common procedures but muck up on the harder or rarer ones. What's needed is for surgeons to regulate themselves and to prevent their colleagues from attempting the complex procedures that they aren't able to do. And resources need to be devoted to improving the existing infrastructure and staffing levels in NHS units rather than funnelling them off to the private sector to create unnecessary competition.

Heart surgeons found out the hard way that you can't defend the indefensible. But until endocrine surgeons follow suit, anyone undergoing thyroid or parathyroid surgery would be well advised to ask how many operations their surgeon does and how his or her results compare to the national average.

PATRICIA HEWITT
May 2005–June 2007

Poor Patsy. Lumbered with the bill for John Reid's spending spree, she had to somehow explain how a health service with record investment could end up in record debt. She came up with some memorable soundbites. 'The NHS has never had it so good' went down so well at the Royal College of Nursing that she was booed and slow hand-clapped by those worried about job cuts. But my favourite quote was: 'A penny wasted in the NHS is a penny stolen from a patient.' This from a government that spent billions on an IT system that hasn't delivered, commercial building contracts that were too secret to scrutinise, sweeteners to open the doors of the NHS to private competition, and management consultants to disguise what was happening from the Labour faithful. Then add in the costs of administrating a continuous and contradictory reform programme. (Establish primary care trusts, then close them down again. Abolish GP fundholding, then build it up again. Build lots of new hospitals then take as much work as possible away from them.) You have to at least admire her brass neck.

Hewitt tried her best to pin the blame on greedy GPs, but it was the Department of Health who had agreed the deal with the consent of Blair and Brown, despite warnings from the BMA negotiators that most GPs would easily hit the targets set for them. Unlike Reid, Hewitt was good with accounts and managed to get the NHS back into the black, causing a lot of resentment and anger on the way. She also had to cop it for the junior doctor job-application fiasco, and paid for it with her own job. No-one loves an accountant, especially one with an accountant's communication skills.

PRIVATE EYE
Don't Believe What You Read

25 August 2005

Should we trust what we read in esteemed medical journals? And are they any good at identifying medical fraud? The answers to both may be 'no', if you believe a recent survey of journal editors carried out by the *BMJ* for the Committee on Publication Ethics. Most journals do not have policies for dealing with misconduct, nor do they have complaints procedures for handling allegations, despite a series of scandalous publications (such as the cloning breakthroughs claimed by Korean scientists).

As Dr Fiona Godlee, editor of the *BMJ*, put it: 'Biomedical journals often have few resources available to them and little in the way of back-up, added to which for many journal editors, the role is part-time. This often makes it very hard for them to pursue matters further. Nevertheless, complaints procedures and guidance for authors should be standard minimum requirements for journals.'

At present, it seems we can't spot the cheats and liars who harm patients and waste money to further their own careers. As Richard Smith, former editor of the *BMJ*, once put it: 'Half of what appears in medical journals is excessive, bent or crummy.' The trouble is, it's hard to spot which half before publication. Smith also believes that medical journals are just an extension of the pharmaceutical industry.[1] Many now carry drug adverts but he does not see this as the main problem. Although it's a clear signal of a journal's financial dependence on the industry, ads are so upfront and conspicuous that they're easy to disregard. Much harder to spot is the bias of industry-sponsored randomised controlled trials: 'Readers see

---

[1] www.plosmedicine.org May 2005; Volume 2 Issue 5.

randomised controlled trials as one of the highest forms of evidence. A large trial published in a major journal has the journal's stamp of approval and may well receive global media coverage. . . . A company will sometimes spend upwards of a million dollars on reprints of the trial.'

Amazingly (or not), studies funded by a company are four times more likely to have results favourable to the company than studies funded from other sources. So how do drug companies manage to get the results they want? The tactics, according to Smith, are numerous. You can conduct a trial of your drug against a treatment known to be inferior. Or trial your drugs against too low a dose of a competitor drug. Or use too high a dose (making the competitor seem toxic). You can use multiple endpoints and just publish the one that's favourable. Or do multi-centre trials ands just publish the favourable centres, or even just publish a subgroup that seems to work.

The bottom line, however, is to construct the trial well enough to get into peer-reviewed journals, which only drug companies have the resources to do. Between two-thirds and three-quarters of the trials published in the major journals are funded by the industry. But if the industry doesn't fund this research, who will? Higher taxes for more publicly funded research. Now there's a vote-winner.

Non-Sexy Illnesses No. 456 – Blackouts

8 September 2005

Around 30% of patients diagnosed with epilepsy actually suffer from a disturbed heart rhythm (arrhythmia), which leads to a temporary loss of consciousness resembling a seizure. Some patients suffer many such attacks of 'reflex syncope' in a short space of time, which is very debilitating and distressing, and yet many go for years without the correct diagnosis or treatment. The lucky few who are diagnosed can be very effectively treated with a pacemaker.

A consultant cardiologist and *Eye* reader describes one such patient who was misdiagnosed with temporal lobe epilepsy for 27 years. She suffered severe bouts of depression and avoided socialising for fear of having an attack. She had to reduce her working week to eighteen hours, was unable to swim alone and received very little help from the NHS.

'Despite her appalling suffering she experienced off-hand treatment at the hands of unmotivated clinicians hiding within a dysfunctional and unresponsive system. Her local neurologist laughed at her, the cardiologist wouldn't deign to see her, and the local commissioner wouldn't agree to her having a pacemaker in London.

'In desperation, she came to me in my private rooms (her GP having refused to refer her to my NHS clinic). I did not charge her. I asked her husband to leave the room, told her to feign a blackout, admitted her to my NHS hospital and put in a pacemaker that afternoon. Since that time she has got a completely new life, with work, friends, exercise and new confidence.'

The consultant, who wishes to remain anonymous, believes the outlook for patients with unsexy illnesses that aren't targeted or given extra resources remains poor. 450 people per million receive pacemakers in the UK for the treatment of slow heart rhythms, compared to an average of 900 in Western Europe. Similarly, only 45 UK patients per million receive implantable cardioverter defibrillators to protect them from sudden cardiac arrest compared to 85 in Western Europe. And France, Germany and Italy also have five times as many electrophysiologists (heart-rate specialists) as the UK.

The top-down, centralist NHS will never be able to treat patients according to clinical need while resources are so unevenly distributed and patients have very little clout in seeking out the treatment they need. Those suffering from recurrent blackouts would be well advised to visit the Syncope Trust and Reflex Anoxic Seizures website (www.stars.org.uk).

The Death of Chest Splitting?

6 October 2005

Do we still need heart surgeons? Most people would rather avoid having their chest split open and with the increasing use of stents to bypass blockages in coronary arteries, UK cardiac surgeons have stopped issuing training numbers because there isn't enough work to go around.

The demise of heart surgery has been predicted ever since angioplasty (dilating blockages with a balloon) arrived in the seventies. Alas, 30% of dilated coronary arteries closed up again soon afterwards and the surgeons stayed in business. The first bare metal stent was inserted in 1986 but once again, a quarter of these blocked at six months.

Drug-eluting stents were developed in the nineties by coating stents with drugs to prevent restenosis. The results so far appear impressive, with reblockage rates down in single figures and cardiologists claiming that 90% of coronary heart disease can now be treated by them, rather than surgeons. Indeed, one cardiologist in the south-west claims to refer just one out of 200 diagnostic angiography cases to surgery. The rest get angioplasty and stents.

Interventional cardiologists (ICs) are also hoping to corner the market in heart attacks, with some research showing that angioplasty and 'hot stenting' shortly afterwards is far more likely to prevent reblockage than the clot-busting drugs currently used. The message – 'if your heart hurts, get to a catheter lab' – will mean a vastly increased, round the clock workload for cardiologists. At present, you only get the gold standard treatment if you have your heart attack in office hours near a specialist centre.

ICs are also taking on the macho, difficult cases (e.g. blockages in the left mainstem coronary artery) previously left to the surgeons. They collect and publish their results on the British Cardiovascular Intervention Society website. Alas, the audit is far from independent (ICs collect their own figures, and enter their own indications, complications and results) but those who do not submit data are at least named and shamed publicly.

ICs also have an unhealthy reliance on the stent industry. The vast majority of research, training and educational meetings is paid for by manufacturers such as Cordis and Boston Scientific and the 'stent wars' competition is fierce with a multi-billion dollar global market. In such an environment, it's easy to see how bias can creep into research and practice.

So how is the NHS coping with the cost of stenting? 52% of stents are currently drug-eluting and the waiting time to see a cardiologist compares well with the rest of Europe. But there have been some almighty cockups. Half of England's 68 catheter labs do diagnosis (angiography) only and have to refer to another centre for treatment (angioplasty). In the new regime of Payment By Results (PBR) they'll become redundant because no-one will pay for the same procedure twice.

Also under PBR, short-stay emergency procedures attract only 40% of the tariff of longer stays, regardless of what it costs the hospital. So brilliant same-day treatment with the best stents gets a fraction of the reimbursement of a cheap bodge-up job over several days. Payment by activity, not outcome, will never improve safety, quality or value for money. Unless the DoH corrects such anomalies, gaming and mediocrity will continue to thrive in the NHS.

Unsexy Illnesses No. 898 – Cystic Fibrosis

17 November 2005

In April 2001, public health minister Yvette Cooper announced a national neonatal screening programme for cystic fibrosis (CF), the UK's most common, life-threatening inherited disease. So why hasn't it happened yet? Biochemical screening for CF has been available in the UK since 1980, and newborns served by laboratories in East Anglia, Trent, Northampton and Leeds have been screened for some years, as have those in Northern Ireland, Wales and Scotland. An England-wide service was due to be rolled out last year, led by the UK Newborn Screening Programme Centre, but four and a half years after Cooper's promise, it still hasn't arrived.

Screening has become more important as treatments for CF have improved. In CF, the lungs and pancreas can get clogged with thick sticky mucous and in the 1930s, when the disease was first recognised, 70% of babies died within a year. Now, thanks to the development of specialist paediatric and adult CF centres, and the combination of early diagnosis and swift treatment, patients can live into their forties.

In the absence of screening, many patients are diagnosed late, if at all. One in 25 of us carry the faulty CF gene, and statistically, there are 2.3 million carriers of the faulty gene and 7,500 people with CF in the UK. However, only 6,000 are currently treated in specialist centres. The remaining 1,500 are either as yet undiagnosed or being treated by non-specialists, who see only a few cases a year and lack the expertise and resources to do it properly. There has been published evidence for seven years that specialist centres get better results,[1] because they treat very aggressively to maintain maximum weight and lung function. However, they cannot reverse the damage done

---

[1] Clinical outcome in relation to care in centres specialising in cystic fibrosis. *British Medical Journal* 1998; 316: 1771–5 (13 June).

by inadequate treatment or late diagnosis. A screening programme that channelled all affected babies into specialist care would help resolve this.

Alas, CF is not a high-priority illness, and research by the CF Trust a year ago found that a third of patients have trouble getting the best drugs and treatments even at specialist centres. Not one of the 38 centres provided 'recommended levels of care', and only nine were able to employ even half the staff they needed. The overall shortfall in funding for CF care was estimated at 50%. At present, indebted PCTs can simply refuse to pay for proper CF care for their patients, which may explain the delay in screening. What's the point in identifying more babies with CF if you aren't going to commit the resources to providing the best treatment?

Meanwhile, £17.5 billion of NHS funding is being put aside for the private sector for absurdly expensive and inflexible PFI contracts and £6.2 billion has been committed to an NHS IT superhighway that has thus far delivered very little. Indeed, according to its boss Richard '£250,000 a year' Granger, it is 'in grave danger of being derailed'. Here's a thought. Give the money back to patients.

Swallow That

9 February 2006
The revelation, courtesy of the Commission for Social Care Inspection, that the elderly are given the wrong drugs in half of all care homes could be construed as progress; when left to their own devices only a third of patients take their tablets properly. This long-standing problem has been compounded of late by the absurd number of pills elderly patients have to pop so GPs can hit the Government's targets and send their children to public school.

Targets do at least concentrate the mind but as Peter

Winocour, a consultant NHS diabetologist puts it: 'targets are often impractical and involve taking too many drugs . . . 10% of type 2 diabetics could require two or three hypoglycaemic agents (ultimately including insulin), at least three antihypertensive agents, two hypolipidaemic agents, and aspirin. A high proportion will also require treatment for coexistent cardiovascular disease and coincidental unrelated chronic disease. It is difficult to see how we can realistically expect patients to comply for long with such a draconian regimen requiring so many separate drugs.'[1]

To illustrate the point, a GP has written to the *Eye* about an elderly woman who was expected to take twenty tablets of sixteen different drugs spaced out over four different time intervals: 'One of the drugs was warfarin, to reduce the risk of stroke, which interacted with a lot of the other drugs and required regular blood tests (INRs) to get the correct dose. However, the INR was wildly variable and we couldn't get the dose of warfarin right. It later transpired that instead of adhering to her absurdly complicated drug regime, she'd tipped all sixteen bottles of tablets into a basket and swallowed twenty at random each day, figuring out it would all even up in the end.'

Given the increasing pill burden of the elderly (as we try to keep them well enough to travel to Switzerland to end their lives), care home staff need more than training to get the tablets right, they need someone with the time to do nothing else all day but dish them out.

[1] Winocour P. Effective diabetes care: a need for realistic targets. *BMJ* 2002; 324: 1577–80.

Moneybags GPs?

19 April 2006

As a GP, I earn £40 an hour. To take home £250,000 a year, as the BBC is suggesting, I'd need to clock up 120 hours a week. I used to do this as a junior doctor, but I was knackered and dangerous. Any GP still putting in those sorts of hours is welcome to the money, although he (and it probably is a he) is also likely to be knackered and dangerous.

This furore over GPs' pay is a convenient smokescreen for Labour's failure to radically improve the NHS. The current debts are not because the reforms are 'biting', but rather because they haven't happened. Getting access to, or time with, the GP you choose is harder than it ever was. And consultations are now driven by targets, not patients.

When I qualified in 1990, I had ten-minute appointments. Today, I still have ten-minute appointments. The patients are equally complicated but more likely to demand and complain (unsurprisingly, given the money going into the NHS). Doctors need time to diagnose and treat safely, patients need it to express themselves, but neither get it. So where's the reform?

As Professor Aidan Halligan, the director of clinical governance for the NHS in England and former deputy chief medical officer put it: 'We have learnt that throwing money at the problem only allows us to do more of what we have always done. Any suggestion of real reform has been a deceit.

'Targets have become an end rather than a means and, together with blinkered performance management, have distorted healthcare priorities. . . . At a moment of unprecedented need, healthcare is suffering a leadership void which has caused it to lose its way.'

Centrally imposed market reforms can never work, not least because the vast majority of the NHS workforce believe health is a right, rather than a commodity. Although GPs, and the drug industry, are earning more for lumbering patients with twenty tablets a day they can't possibly remember to take, the vast majority of NHS funding still goes into hospitals. The Tories allowed some GPs to develop better community services (and higher wages) through fundholding, but it was an iniquitous system that penalised patients of non-fundholders. However the ethos of providing cheaper, better care for patients outside hospitals was correct.

Alas Labour, having preached the evils of fundholding in opposition, could not draw on its strengths and extend it to all. So it was abolished. Now, nine years later, fundholding has been resurrected as practice-based commissioning, but now all the new money has been gobbled up (largely by hospitals) and the NHS is rife with debt, panic and job insecurity. In such a climate, it can only fail.

For nine years, Blair's main focus has been on waiting times for hospital treatment, which were eighteen months when he took over and which he hopes will be eighteen weeks when he leaves. This would be an undoubted improvement, at huge cost, but given that over 90% of healthcare has nothing to do with hospitals, it hardly represents system reform. Instead, we've had nine years lurching between contradictory initiatives and – surprise, surprise – we've hardly moved at all. Time to blame those greedy GPs.

Placebos For All

1 June 2006
The exhortation of thirteen senior consultants that the NHS should desist from funding unproven alternative therapies (*The Times*, May 23) was a touch biased, given that many conventional treatments are also of dubious benefit. According to *Clinical Evidence* (www.clinicalevidence.com), only 15% of the thousands of treatments they have reviewed have been

proven to be beneficial. A further 23% are likely to be beneficial, 7% are a trade-off between benefits and harms, 5% are unlikely to be beneficial, 4% are likely to be ineffective or harmful and a whopping 46% are of 'unknown effectiveness'. Clearly, much more research needs to be funded before the NHS can claim to be evidence-based.

Surgery is impossible to subject to the gold standard 'double-blind randomised controlled trial' since any surgeon worth his salt knows if he is performing a proper or sham operation. But the placebo effect is just as evident in surgery as it is in homeopathy. Patients with osteoarthritis who are tricked into thinking their knee joint has been washed out and the bits removed have as much pain reduction and improved movement as those who've had proper arthroscopy.[1] For decades, orthopaedic surgeons have earned a fortune just by blowing air into joints.

There is no doubt that the vast majority of complementary therapies also operate on the placebo effect. In the few trials where acupuncture or homeopathy have been shown to work, it doesn't much matter what remedy you give or where you stick the needles. What matters is the strength of the relationship between therapist and client, and the belief, expectation and suggestion that goes with it. One reason it costs drug companies nearly a billion dollars to get a new drug to market is the great difficulty many of them have in out-performing a placebo.

Placebos produce noticeable improvements across a whole range of symptoms and illnesses, such as pain, tiredness, nausea, high blood pressure, angina, asthma, hay fever, headaches, PMT, depression, anxiety, peptic ulcers, high cholesterol, insomnia, hot flushes and social problems. They can reduce the frequency of epileptic seizures, have nasty side-effects and

---

[1] Moseley et al. *New England Journal of Medicine* 2002; 347: 81–8.

reverse the effects of powerful drugs. Placebos even work if you tell patients that's what they're taking. In one study,[2] fifteen psychiatric patients suffering from neurotic symptoms were told: 'We feel that a so-called sugar pill may help you. Do you know what a sugar pill is? A sugar pill is a pill with no medicine in it at all. I think this pill will help you as it has helped so many others. Are you willing to try this pill?' Fourteen said yes and thirteen improved during the week, some a great deal, including one previously suicidal patient.

All medicine is in large part placebo, yet some doctors are jealous of the complementary therapists' freedom to 'big up' their placebo effect by talking unscientific bollocks. But far from wasting money, complementary therapy does in many cases save it by avoiding the prescription of more expensive, and potentially harmful drugs. In a free-at-the-front-door health service, patients flood in with all manner of bizarre symptoms and emotional hang-ups that science has yet to find an answer for. Without complementary therapy, patients end up on Prozac or painkillers just to get them out of the door.

The only other alternative is counselling, which has some evidence base but it's used by GPs to pass the buck. As Dr Phil Peverley puts it: 'Our referral letters essentially say the same thing: "Dear counsellor, I don't want to talk to this patient any more. You do it." . . . Our counsellor was a proper nurse until three months ago, but she is now trained to listen to any old shite without laughing.'[3]

Alas, I can't practise complementary therapy without laughing ('you've got too much jitsu in your tsubo . . .') but I know plenty of people who can. The NHS would implode without them.

[2] Park L, Covi L. Non blind Placebo Trial. *Archives of General Psychiatry* 1965; 12: 336–45.
[3] Peverley. *Pulse Magazine* 1 June 2006.

Regulating Doctors

26 July 2006

What's the best way to regulate doctors? No-one seems to know, least of all the chief medical officer Liam Donaldson. His post-Shipman review (*Good Doctors, Safer Patients*), is full of the same rhetoric as its post-Bristol predecessor (*Supporting Doctors, Protecting Patients*), and its scatter-gun approach of 44 recommendations could just add a hugely expensive 'scrutiny bureaucracy' without making doctors better or patients safer.

Donaldson's most contentious suggestion is for the burden of proof in actions against doctors to be lowered from criminal ('beyond reasonable doubt') to civil ('on the balance of probability'). This may pick up doctors who are dangerous for patients but not too dangerous for the GMC, but it may also result in mass suspensions and a surge in defensive medicine where doctors over-investigate and refer rather than take the buck themselves. This would be extremely expensive and counter to the Government's aim of getting GPs to accept more responsibility and minimise hospital care.

Donaldson also wants doctors to be re-licensed every five years, rather than just once on qualification and never again thereafter. This sounds reasonable, and indeed I underwent a form of re-licensing last year when I returned to general practice after a career break. It consisted of a knowledge-based multiple choice questionnaire (MCQ), two hours of video consultations and a structured trainer's report. I passed, but then again the tests are hard to fail. The MCQ is positively marked, so a monkey with a pencil would get 50% by chance alone. The video does not have to be continuous, so you can exclude any consultation where you've cocked up badly. And trainers have a habit of passing their trainees, lest it reflect badly on their teaching.

What matters is not whether doctors can jump through the

artificial hoops of exams (most can, which is how we became doctors in the first place) but whether the consequences of our everyday actions lead to avoidable harm for patients. The most useful scrutiny I have had is the analysis of my actions by other doctors, particularly the cockups and near misses. For example, I recently diagnosed a patient's chest pain as non-cardiac, based on the history. Four months later, he had a heart attack.

Like any other doctor, I want to know if I got it wrong and, if so, what I should do to get it right next time. Most GP practices and hospitals have regular significant-event audit meetings; some are rigorous and at times brutal, but others tend to be too uncritical for fear of upsetting colleagues. What's needed are doctors in every region, who are independent of the medical establishment, to analyse potential errors in a fair and balanced way. Both doctors and patients would then get quick, impartial feedback. And those doctors who repeatedly err would be picked up earlier.

I first argued for an independent medical inspectorate focusing on errors in 1999.[1] Sir Liam's answer is to introduce local, medically qualified 'GMC affiliates', paired with a public buddy. But without true independence, it seems no more likely to succeed than the 'Assessment and Support Centres' he proposed seven years ago.

Politicians don't trust doctors to regulate themselves in secret, but neither do doctors trust politicians or the GMC to do it fairly and competently. The key question is 'Who picks up doctors' mistakes?' If it's done independently, swiftly and fairly, we'll all benefit. If it becomes a political process, where good doctors are defined as those who do what Labour wants them to, it'll be a disaster.

[1] See Pickering W. in *Regulating Doctors*. ISBN 1–903–386–0

There's Only Four NHSs

26 July 2006

During the last election, Tony Blair took the piss out of the Welsh health service for its long waiting times compared to England. Given that Wales is theoretically served by the same National Health Service that Blair had promised to turn around it seemed a brave call, and one that caused huge embarrassment to Welsh Labour MPs. But the Welsh Assembly has chosen to take their NHS in a different direction to Blair's relentless focus on competition and privatisation in England. In Wales, the emphasis is on tackling the causes of ill health, rather than trying to micromanage the NHS. So who'll have the last laugh?

Instead of spending hundreds of millions of pounds abolishing community health councils, setting up a Commission for Public and Patient Involvement in Health and closing it down again, Wales simply kept the CHCs. It has invested in free breakfasts for primary school children and free prescriptions for all. Devolved parliament in Scotland has funded free personal care for the elderly, whereas in England thousands of elderly patients are denied nursing care on the NHS because their medical needs are artificially reclassified as 'social' and they have to sell their homes to pay for care.

The Scottish Parliament also managed to reconfigure its health services with broad support from the public and health service staff, in marked contrast to the divisive battles over privatisation that the English NHS is enduring. In Wales and Scotland, the ethos is more to trust professionals to do their jobs out of a sense of vocation, rather than rely on market forces and excessive regulation to do it for them. PCTs, payment by results, star ratings, compulsory choice and practice-based commissioning do not even exist in Wales or Scotland. And the hugely bureaucratic raft of proposals that Sir Liam Donaldson introduced to revalidate doctors only applies to England.

The downside for Wales and Scotland is that their left-wing, increasingly nationalist approach has ducked the politically combustible issue of hospital closures. In Wales, the mindset is that each area should offer uniform services, which is neither efficient nor cost-effective. In Northern Ireland hospital activity is 26% lower than England per bed. Scotland is using the private sector to get waiting lists down, though much less so than England and only when there is a real need (as opposed to the English stance of competition for the hell of it).

Scotland's reform programme seems to be the most co-ordinated, with its focus on networks and partnerships. In Wales, first minister Rhodri Morgan is aiming for 'clear red water' between Cardiff and London and the Lib Dems are too supine to object. In England, the volume and haste of new initiatives, some of which directly contradict others, has meant that not even senior managers are clear about what they're supposed to be aiming for.

What is clear is that there is no UK focus in health policy, and there are huge disparities in entitlement and treatment across four countries. This is completely contrary to the notions of equity and treatment according to need, and it'll be some years before we discover who got it right. The three smaller countries at least have the advantage of watching the English NHS crash and burn, and then cherry-picking the good bits. In the meantime, go to England for quick operations, Wales for free prescriptions, Scotland for long-term care and Northern Ireland if you don't like change.

Indiscreet Doctors

7 September 2006
Would you let someone who claims to be a doctor examine you, without any pretence of privacy, on a crowded high street?

And let it be filmed? Fortunately for the makers of *Street Doctors* (*The One Show*, BBC1, September 4–8), there are plenty of people who will. But can you give informed consent to a televised medical ambush?

My worst experience of this was presenting *As it Happens* for Channel 4, live from City Hospital in 1997. The producer was desperate to film cardiac resuscitation, and reckoned he could get consent too: 'We'll put a two-minute delay on the filming and if the resuscitation's successful, we'll get the patient to sign the release form when he comes round.' Mercifully, it never happened.

A year later, BBC1 released the *Human Body*, fronted by Robert Winston, which managed to get a dying man to consent to filming his death, a BBC researcher to consent to thermal imaging of his erect penis and pregnant women awaiting terminations to consent to intra-uterine filming of foetal development.

In 2002, BBC3 pushed the boundaries further with *Sex, Warts and All*, a much praised series on sexual health which somehow got patients to admit to having sexually transmitted infections and to show their genitals (warts and all) to the camera. As adviser Dr Rak Nandwani put it, 'It's had a great impact in reducing the stigma of sexual health clinics, and has encouraged people to attend.'

Destigmatisation is the standard defence of all medical confession programmes, but rarely is much thought given to the consequences of such public exposure. On *Street Doctors*, a man at a fruit and veg market was found to have a blood pressure of 188/109, which is certainly worth knowing about. But do you want to share it with your employer or insurer?

In 2004, I was asked to comment on the health of the 'volunteers' for BBC1's *Fat Nation*, filmed live from a street in Birmingham. The producer had assembled a spreadsheet of coronary risk factors (blood pressure, cholesterol, smoking and diabetic status) that the inhabitants had apparently consented to having read out on BBC1 when signing their release forms. The results were so shocking, with half the street likely to suffer a heart attack or worse in the next decade, that the item was dropped because it didn't fit in with the happy clappy 'let's get fit together' ethos.

Back on *Street Doctor*, fruit and veg man is told his blood pressure is '8 out of 10' on a scale of badness, whatever that means. Another woman is told she might have rheumatoid arthritis as she leans on her burger bar and a boy is undressed to find he has 'molluscum contagiosum' under his arm: 'Nothing to worry about,' claims Doctor Barbara, though whether he'll see it that way in the playground the morning after transmission is debatable.

Inevitably, a man takes his trousers off and squats on a bag of shallots to be examined, but even more undignified was a man lying on a mat with his head resting on the kerb. Most of what gets dished out is reassurance, but medicine has a habit of dishing out nasty surprises and examining a pregnant woman in the middle of Bury market would be disastrous if the foetal heartbeat was absent.

The GMC and BMA agree on very few things, but patient confidentiality is one of them. Bizarrely, one of the street doctors is George Rae, who in July came second in a vote to become chairman of the BMA and is now wandering around Manchester exhorting patients to strip off in public and 'worry yourself not'. Come back Frankie Howerd.

Doctors and the Drug Industry

6 October 2006

Does the drug industry still have too much influence over doctors? I was asked to support this motion, with Labour MP Howard Stoate, at the Oxford Union last month. The debate was paid for by the industry and attended by its employees, so unsurprisingly we lost. But I left £500 richer (plus expenses, meal and overnight accommodation).

Opposing us were two GPs, Peter Fellows and George 'street doctor' Rae, current and former Chairmen of the BMA prescribing sub-committee. Their (paraphrased) argument is that medicine is now so closely scrutinised and regulated, with prescribing largely dictated by evidence-based formularies, that it's far harder for doctors to wander off-message and prescribe bucket-loads of an unproven drug because they like the breasts of a cheerleader rep. Besides, doctors are professionals who are trained to absorb any amount of excessive hospitality without it clouding our professional judgement.

Indeed, the days of excessive hospitality are supposed to be over, thanks to the new Association of the British Pharmaceutical Industry (ABPI) code that came into effect on January 1, 2006. Freebies given to doctors, otherwise known as promotional aids, should cost no more than £6 (excluding VAT). This should be the street value, so a company can't bulk buy 20,000 rubber nun suits with 'Pfizer' tattooed above the buttocks if I can't buy the same item in my local corner shop for £6 or less.

Also, the gift has to be relevant to professional practice. Branded thermos flasks, travel rugs, teapots, dentures, barometers etc. are out. And the gift has to be matched to the recipient. For example, a rep can't give a receptionist a tongue depressor (even if she's really earned one). Travel expenses can't be paid for local meetings and all flights are economy only (unless you're a speaker). You can't take your wife, lover or children unless there's a good professional reason for it. There are dozens more rules ranging from the size of the lettering on 'laminated leave pieces' to the format of the inane adverts placed in medical journals. And unlike medical self-regulation, where very few people shop a colleague, competitors are lining up to report you if you stray from the code.

The downside is that membership of the ABPI isn't compulsory, and given that most doctors haven't got a clue who's in and who's out, suspension seems only to cause a little internal embarrassment. On February 10, 2006, Abbott Laboratories were suspended from the ABPI for 'a minimum of six months' after being rumbled taking doctors on various corporate jollies (one to Wimbledon and two to a greyhound racing stadium). However, it was the escort of a doctor to an evening presentation with two leading-edge female presenters (i.e. a lap-dancing bar) that raised the most eyebrows.

Abbott don't seem to have suffered commercially for their slapped wrist and indeed they were reinstated to the ABPI on July 1, less than five months into their minimum six-month suspension. Overall, the drug industry in the UK spends £1.65 billion marketing its drugs, whereas the Department of Health spends just £4.5 million a year providing independent prescribing information to doctors (or at least it did until it axed its subscription to the excellent *Drugs and Therapeutics Bulletin*). Drug companies pay for or subsidise just about every educational meeting doctors attend. They wouldn't do it without some return.

One solution would be for doctors to pay for their own education, or at least for the industry to pool its educational grants so no individual company has undue influence over training. But all this is pointless if we can't trust the 'evidence' on which our training is based. The drug industry is certainly clearing up its front-of-house operations, but companies still control the research and information flow about their own products, and they use medical journals as an extension of their marketing arm. If all companies were obliged to pool their clinical-research funding, so that all large-scale trials could be performed and published independently of the manufacturer, we'd all be a lot safer.

Statins for All?

20 October 2006

Should you try to get your cholesterol as low as possible? What you eat has very little bearing on your blood level of 'bad cholesterol' (LDL), so the only way to reduce it is to take statins. This would certainly please the pharmaceutical industry, which already makes more than £20 billion a year on this class of drug, but is anyone swallowing it?

Statins are the biggest-selling drugs ever, and by inhibiting an enzyme involved in the liver synthesis of cholesterol, they reduce the level of circulating cholesterol in the bloodstream. If you already have heart disease, or lots of risk factors for it (diabetes, high blood pressure, smoking), there is good evidence that statins reduce your risk of 'future cardiac events'. It's assumed they do this by stopping the build-up of rancid LDL in the walls of your arteries but some studies show they cut the risk of heart disease independently of their effect on cholesterol. However they work, they reduce the risk of nasty things happening to your heart. The key questions are which patients should take a statin and how much?

In the UK, GPs are 'incentivised' (i.e. bribed) by the Government to get the total cholesterol of patients with heart disease and stroke (or at 30% risk of having either in the next decade), down to 5 mmol/l or less. This doesn't make much sense, since you need to know how much of it is good (HDL) or bad (LDL) but these tests are more expensive so we lump it all together. As a result, two and a half million UK patients are already on statins, at an average annual cost of over £150 each. GPs get their payments if they get 60% of their patients to target. Some patients, particularly those at much higher risk with very high cholesterol levels, are harder to treat but provided a GP has ticked off the easy 60%, there's no financial incentive to treat the patients who need it most.

Recently, the Joint British Societies have recommended a target total cholesterol of 4 mmol/l and an LDL of less than 2 mmol/l in high-risk groups. The US National Cholesterol Program recommends an even tougher target of 1.81 mmol/l. This would mean far more patients on more statins, a situation that the NHS can't afford, so GP targets are likely to remain unchanged.

The vast majority of men in the UK, and a substantial minority of women, have an LDL above 1.81 mmol/l but most are at low risk of heart disease and shouldn't go anywhere near a statin. Alas, the aggressive promotion of the link between cholesterol and heart disease and the availability of over-the-counter statins has meant that a lot more lower-risk patients are taking drugs they don't need to. A major study conducted among healthy Scots (yes, there are a few) found that if 10,000 people took statins for five years, 9,755 would receive no benefit. They would all, however, suffer from the medical dependency of lifelong medication and some would get unpleasant (and rarely, very serious) side-effects.

Statins are of huge benefit to those at high risk of heart disease, and no use, or even harmful, to those at low risk. But, like blood pressure medicines, they only work if you take them for life and this is where it all starts to fall apart. The majority of patients on statins either stop taking the drug altogether or take less than the prescribed dose within a year. In the long term, only a third of patients take them effectively. Instead of toughening up the targets and extending the net to create more cholesterol patients, we should concentrate our efforts on those at highest risk and make their tablet taking as simple, low-dose and side-effect-free as possible. Of the £20 billion spent globally on statins, up to £14 billion could already be wasted on patients who refuse to take them. Surely not a time to prescribe more.

Reconfiguration

2 November 2006

Why has Labour failed to win the hearts and minds of doctors for its reform programme? For a while it won their silence, by stuffing their mouths with gold and cutting waiting times for surgery. But last week, in the fag end of Blair's administration, hundreds of members of the most politically apathetic profession donned catchy 'Working for a better NHS' scarves and marched on parliament, mumbling 'NHS SOS'.

There is a groundswell of opinion amongst doctors that the Government has badly screwed up its '£100 billion a year' chance to save the NHS, at least in England. Its biggest error has been to become so preoccupied with attracting private business that it has neglected to reconfigure the NHS until hospitals are deeply in debt. So even rational decisions about which hospitals and services need to close or merge for safety reasons are clouded in protests about finance and privatisation. Add in the political sensibilities of closures in marginal constituencies, and the most important reform is doomed to failure.

Since exposing the Bristol cardiac disaster in 1992, I have argued that specialist, hi-tech services have to be centralised in fewer centres where resources are concentrated and there is a sufficient caseload for safe training and meaningful audit. The *Eye* has exposed a succession of scandals where surgeons were doing highly complex operations occasionally, and often badly, and successfully campaigned for children's liver surgery and cleft palate repair to be restricted to fewer, accredited centres.

As technology has advanced over the last fifteen years, and the European working time directive kicked in, the centralisation argument has applied to more specialties. There are too many district general hospitals in the NHS and too many small casualty departments and paediatric units. This was evident when Labour took office and if they'd used the goodwill of the initial cash injection to get NHS staff and patients to agree on how local services needed to change, they might have succeeded.

Instead they threw the money at ill-conceived PFI deals, private surgical contractors, pointless quangos, the destruction of GP fundholding, the creation of 300 PCTs, the destruction of half of the PCTs and the reintroduction of GP fundholding. The attempt to introduce market competition and get money to follow the patient kicked off with a disastrous tariff system that didn't compensate hospitals for the risk and complexity of their work and led to record debts and the resignation of the chief executive, Nigel Crisp. The 2007–08 tariff has just been announced, and trusts will have to spend an enormous amount of time trying to 'unbundle it' (i.e. fight with each other to make sure they get paid for all their bits of treatment).

As in America, a hospital's survival will become entirely dependent on the success of its coding and debt collection departments, which are a hugely expensive, administrative cash drain. Contrast this to the tariff-free NHS in Scotland, which is well down the road of reconfiguration thanks to a clear national plan, extensive parliamentary debate, cross-party support and the involvement of staff and patients. Markets and fragmentation don't work in healthcare; consultation and co-operation do. Alas, it's too late for the English NHS.

NICE Rationing

12 December 2006
It's not often that a front-bench MP admits that rationing in the NHS exists, and has to exist, so hats off to shadow health secretaries Andrew Lansley (Con) and Steve Webb (Lib Dem). Admittedly I put the words in their mouths, but they repeated them without much prompting.

The occasion was the National Institute for Health and

Clinical Excellence (NICE) conference, which I was paid to chair (though an assessment of my value for money is pending). Representing Labour was GP/MP Howard Stoate, who wouldn't admit to rationing but made up for it by declaring that the Government's reform programme was too quick and in the wrong order. Alas, he's unlikely to become health secretary.

NICE exists to try to make the rationing of healthcare rational. After lengthy analysis of the evidence, it approves most treatments but gets a good media kicking for taking its time to reach a judgement (Herceptin) or deciding which treatments shouldn't be funded by the NHS (Alzheimer's drugs in early dementia, Velcade for myeloma).

The result is a covert system of co-payments, where the rich top up their NHS treatment with private prescriptions for non-NICE approved drugs. This, according to Professor Karol Sikora, is happening throughout the NHS. So what's to stop cancer specialists offering private patients expensive new drugs that only add a few months to life? Their conscience, apparently.

But Labour's health reforms are not evaluated with the same rigour as new treatments. If Patsy Hewitt really wants to convince the public about NHS reconfiguration, she needs to publish detailed service planning and a rationale which can be supported by evidence. Alas, all she has is ideology. Crippling hospitals with PFI debts and throwing money at ISTCs to cherry-pick easy operations has no evidence base, other than the splintered, debt-ridden service it has spawned.

The most compelling evidence that the health reforms have failed is that, under Blair, the gap between rich and poor has widened. The UK has one of the most unequal societies in Europe and every one of Labour's solutions has inadvertently made it worse. Waiting-list initiatives and patient-choice programmes favour the well-educated, who are also more likely to read and act on NICE guidelines. This isn't all Labour's fault;

there's an inherent bias amongst NHS staff, especially doctors, to favour patients who are more like ourselves.

In contrast, poorer patients are less likely to access good preventative care and routine surgery, and hence very reliant on the very emergency services which Labour are closing. The provision of healthcare has always been poor where the need is greatest, and excluding the obese and smokers from treatment, as is happening in some areas, will widen the gap further. Poorer patients often have more than one illness and the window of opportunity for treatment is narrow. If Labour was really concerned about equality, it would prioritise treatment on the basis of postcode so the poor get treated more quickly than the rich. And it would reinstate a properly funded public health specialty to evaluate its reforms. As Professor Rod Griffiths told the conference: 'The poor aren't "hard to reach". The tobacco industry and drug pushers have no problem reaching them. It's just that the politicians and the NHS don't want to.'

Choose and Book Balls

26 December 2006

In September 2005, 78-year-old *Eye* reader Gordon Beare had a knee operation. This made one leg shorter than the other, necessitating orthopaedic shoes to level them up. Until recently, his GP would have organised referral to the orthotic department of his local hospital but under the new system of Choose and Book, Mr Beare has to organise his own referral by phoning up the Clinical Assessment Service (01296 710986 between 9.00 and 17.00 Monday to Friday excluding public holidays). He then has to choose one of fifteen units on offer and quote his unique booking reference number (0000–9236–9596) and unique computer-generated password ('cake counter').

If he prefers, he can book over the internet at www.nhs.uk/healthspace and select 'choose and book'. However, he needs to be careful entering his password to put a space between 'cake' and 'counter'. If he doesn't like 'cake counter' he can go back to his GP and ask for it to be changed, or he can do it over the phone (0845 60 88 88 8), via text phone (0845 8 50 22 50) or internet (see above).

More important for Mr Beare is to know which of the fifteen units makes the best orthopaedic shoes but, alas, he is given no information as to the competence of the shoe-makers. He was also given no information about getting transport to and from any of the fifteen units, a pressing concern for someone with unequal legs. So, he phoned up and opted for his nearest unit (Colchester) who offered him a choice of two appointments six weeks apart, but was told to contact his GP about arranging transport.

His GP no longer arranges transport and he was given a number to ring (01206 742354) which he thinks might be an ambulance service but in any case couldn't offer him transport as he was outside of their area. As Mr Beare or Cake space Counter, as he is now known, puts it: 'Should I give up? Is it all a dream? At 78 I don't want all this aggro.'

Neither, it appears, do many doctors. GPs have an ethical and legal duty to refer patients to safe, high-quality services but neither they, nor their patients, are given any meaningful outcome data on which to base their choice. In the old system, consultants could prioritise patients referred to them, but under Choose and Book, it's up to the GP to prioritise the problem, which he or she may not feel able to do. An investigation by *Pulse* magazine found that electronic referrals do not always arrive in time for the appointment, or can't be opened, and that referral management centres are cancelling or diverting referrals deemed inappropriate.

Jeremy Fairbank, a consultant at the Nuffield Orthopaedic

Centre NHS Trust, described the system as 'complex, expensive and unworkable'. Jonathan Edwards, a professor at University College London, is having 'every possible problem'. Dr Paul Reilly, a rheumatologist at Frimley Park Hospital in Surrey, claimed preferential treatment given to C&B patients meant 'trivial problems are seen ahead of serious ones.' And Dr Mark Pugh on the Isle of Wight has given up on the screening software as 'it is a pain in the arse to use.'

To be fair, some GPs, such as Labour MP Howard Stoate, positively enjoy using Choose and Book, but the over-complicated transfer of power and responsibility to patients without adequate information or engagement of doctors could lead to depersonalisation, discontent and disaster. And it's no way to get a pair of orthopaedic shoes.

More GP Balls

26 January 2007
There are few sights less edifying in the NHS than Patricia Hewitt's brass neck, and it reached goitrous proportions with her latest attack on 'greedy, lazy' GPs. By committing the heinous crime of hitting all their targets and delivering precisely what their government-negotiated contract asked of them, they are guilty of bankrupting the NHS. Right.

Contrast this with the contracts offered to private companies to take over NHS diagnostics and surgery. These were guaranteed (i.e. paid whether patients were seen or not), paid above the going rate and allowed the cherry-picking of easy cases while leaving the NHS to mop up any cockups or act as a sink for patients too sick to turn a profit. Despite all these advantages, many companies have failed to treat their target volume of patients.

Doctors have also voiced concerns about the quality of care

provided in Independent Sector Treatment Centres (ISTCs). This was dismissed by the Government as protectionist scaremongering but on the day Hewitt went for the GPs' jugular, the Healthcare Commission announced that the data on the clinical quality of ISTCs was 'incomplete and of extremely poor quality'. So what's the story? GPs fulfilling their contracts and collecting their payments, or expensive, unfair, under-performing and unaudited private treatment centres?

The healthy sums paid to GP partners were entirely predictable. Dangle a big carrot in front of intelligent, ambitious small businesses and it tends to get eaten. Unlike ISTCs, GPs have now contributed a huge amount of data to be entered into the NHS IT programme, should it ever deliver on its (under-performing, hugely overspent) contract. What's harder to assess is whether the GP contract will radically improve patient care and provide value for money. There are early signs that diabetic care is improving, and perhaps the care for patients with heart disease and stroke, but it's hard to prove because there was very little comparative data prior to the contract.[1]

Removing out-of-hours obligations from GPs and carving general practice up into targets is merely a way of introducing privatisation. The blame heaped on GPs for doing what was asked of them will further fuel the argument for more competition. Companies who have saturated the healthcare market in their own countries are using the NHS as a gateway to Europe, waved in by Labour. The Government recently published its NHS Operating Framework, which makes an interesting comparison to the ten core principles that they set out in the 2000 NHS Plan. Seven years ago, they pledged that 'Public funds for healthcare will be devoted solely to NHS patients.' This pledge has now been quietly shelved, as public

---

[1] www.gpcontract.co.uk

funds for healthcare are increasingly devoted to the shareholders of private companies.

The latest game is to privatise outpatients by littering the country with Capture Assess Treat and Support (CATS) centres. Patients referred to hospital will be caught in Netcare's net whether they chose to be or not. White-elephant PFI-indebted hospitals won't be able to compete and will try to cannibalise surrounding hospitals, which are already running over capacity. And demand from an ageing population will rise year on year. The latest delusion is that transferring hospital services to GPs with special interests is cheaper (it isn't) and will reduce demand. The more you train GPs, the more they realise what is possible and the more they refer to hospital. The NHS is heading for meltdown and once again, it'll all be the GPs' fault.

Doctors Not To Be

8 March 2007
Are the careers of eight thousand junior doctors being stuffed up on purpose? The rushed implementation of the Modernising Medical Careers (MMC) programme looks like just another Labour cockup, but its consequences are suspiciously advantageous to a Government intent on busting the medical cabal.

The failure of the Medical Training Application Service (MTAS), a centrallycontrolled computerised bun fight, was predictable to anyone with a passing knowledge of NHS IT programmes. It was flawed in its content, an unvalidated bullshitters' paradise that has allowed erudite disaster-zones to get jobs at the expense of much better doctors, and flawed in its delivery. Making so many doctors apply at the same time was bound to lead to persistent crashing of the site, lost applications, interviews offered for specialities not even applied for and interviews at both ends of the country on the same day.

The Government has been able to ignore earlier concerns that the new system was unfair and unworkable, safe in the knowledge that doctors are finding it hard to get public sympathy. Greedy GPs and consultants, rather than privatisation and target-chasing, have been cleverly fingered as the prime cause of NHS debt, and junior doctors bleating to the media that they may have to become lawyers, work in the City or move to Australia will have Patsy Hewitt chuckling in her cornflakes. The shit has finally reached the fan, thanks to West Midlands surgeons suspending their junior appointments, but health minister Lord Hunt was unfazed: 'MMC was devised with the help and support of the Royal Colleges, the Academy of Medical Sciences and the BMA.' So it's all their fault.

But what's in it for Labour? Having acknowledged they were stuffed by the BMA over consultant and GP contracts, the Government – having increased doctors' numbers – now wants to get by with as few as possible. Doctors have priced themselves out of the market, so medicine is being broken down into simplistic tasks that can be hived off to private companies employing lowest common denominator health workers. Having 30,000 junior doctors compete for 22,000 jobs creates sufficient anxiety and insecurity for those with a job to work illegal hours covering holes in the NHS without whistleblowing.

Junior doctors aren't going down without a fight (support them at www.remedyuk.org) but is seems unlikely that enough would resign en masse to panic the Government. A more likely scenario is that they'll cancel their memberships of the BMA and Royal Colleges, a situation that would delight Labour. The GMC has already been stuffed by Liam Donaldson's ludicrously bureaucratic re-licensing plans, and taking out the rest of the medical establishment would make doctors even easier to control.

The Department of Health has announced a review of

MTAS, but not suspended it. Thousands of juniors have joined up as RemedyUK, and are planning a protest on March 17 from the Royal College of Physicians to the Royal College of Surgeons. But to get public and media support, doctors need to explain how their personal misfortune will affect patients.

For the NHS to thrive, it has to ensure the best and brightest doctors are given the right jobs. MTAS doesn't appear capable of ensuring this. When I'm finally dragged kicking and screaming into an NHS ward, I want to be treated by a doctor with sufficient wisdom, skill and motivation to do the job properly, not a dumbed-down generic health worker reading from a guideline. Cutting down the supply of good doctors may well balance the NHS books in time to save Hewitt, but the long-term consequences will be dire for patient safety.

Cancer Jabs

22 March 2007

Have you taken your daughter for a cervical cancer jab yet? I've yet to be asked for it by any parent, but I know several doctors who've vaccinated their daughters against human papilloma virus types 16 and 18, which cause 70% of cervical cancers. One has vaccinated her sons too, on the back of a *Lancet* editorial that argued all adolescents should be immunised against HPV.[1] This would prevent men passing on these cancerous strains to unvaccinated women, and the vaccine (Gardasil) has the added bonus of protecting against HPV types 6 and 11, which cause 90% of genital warts. Having spent hours in a stuffy clinic trying to freeze them off, I'm sure this would be a huge bonus all round.

Not everyone agrees. Dr Angela Raffle, a public health specialist who oversees cervical screening in the Bristol area,

---

[1] *Lancet* 7 October 2006.

described the editorial as 'disastrous for public health. Countries with high mortality and no screening can achieve major benefit from vaccination. But rushed implementation in Europe will undermine existing cervical screening – which already averts 80% of cervical cancer deaths – and leave women less protected than now.'[2]

True, girls who've been vaccinated might not bother to have cervical screening in later life. The vaccine only protects against 70% of cases of cervical cancer and it's not yet clear how long the protection lasts for. So cervical screening would still be needed to check the effectiveness of the vaccine and pick up the 30% of cancers that aren't covered. However, screening itself is no picnic – minor smear changes cause considerable anxiety and later stage pre-cancerous changes are unpleasant to treat with significant side-effects.

If the vaccine works as well as the manufacturers (Sanofi Pasteur MSD) say it does, the side-effects of screening would be greatly reduced since, as well as protecting against cancer, it should also reduce smear abnormalities at all stages. After the Vioxx scandal, some doctors are reluctant to trust data presented by MSD. But the safety and efficacy information have seen Gardasil get a licence in over 40 countries and it seems unlikely that an 'empty shell' vaccine, with no genetic viral material in it, could pose significant risks.

A bigger challenge is convincing the tabloids of the wisdom of vaccinating pre-teen girls and getting the cash-strapped NHS to foot the bill for a national immunisation plan. The immune response to the vaccine is better if it is given at an early age. No-one suggests that the rubella jab encourages girls to have sex, but the knowledge that cervical cancer is caused by a sexually transmitted infection has turned HPV vaccination into a red-top 'sex jab for schoolgirls'.

---

[2] *Lancet* letters 3 February 2007.

Immunisation programmes are up and running in the US, Australia and several European countries but Labour's plan to introduce immunisation for girls in their first year at secondary school looks like missing the boat this September. The decision was supposed to be announced by the Joint Committee on Vaccination and Immunisation in January, but now seems destined to be delayed until at least June, too late to introduce for the start of the school year. This may just be traditional British scepticism, but the record NHS debts don't help and one DoH source has suggested Gordon Brown wants to make the announcement himself, on becoming a 'woman-friendly' twinkle-toothed premier. Quite how friendly this would be to girls who miss out on protection for the sake of political expediency is unclear. In the meantime, the vaccine is only available privately (£241.50 for three injections plus labour) or from a brave GP prepared to risk the wrath of the PCT.

Junior Doctor Job Fiasco (continued)

30 April 2007
Ever wanted to be a doctor? Couldn't get the grades? Well now you don't have to. Just log onto the MTAS website and you can access the personal details of hundreds of junior doctors. Why do medicine the hard way when you can become a doctor overnight with identity fraud?

This laughable security lapse in the on-line job application software for doctors and medical students has now been fixed . . . but only by taking down the whole site. So, with just thirteen weeks to go before August 1, junior doctors can't get any details of where and when their interviews are. But health minister Lord Hunt was wheeled out to assure us that 'top security advisers' from 'expert external companies' were looking at the lapses as a matter of urgency (and public cost).

Most disturbing was not the leaking of the sexual orientation and religion of named doctors (given the record of IT in the NHS, this was to be expected) but that such a spreadsheet existed in the first place. Such details should only ever be collected anonymously to ensure lack of discrimination, not attributed to named individuals when the only result can be to increase discrimination. So the Modernising Medical Careers programme may now face legal challenges for breaching confidentiality, as well as being incompetent and unfair.

Hunt tried to put the initial lapse down to a malicious leak, and then 'teething problems'. But when it emerged that junior doctors could easily hack into each other's job applications and change them if they so desired, it became apparent that the whole programme was unsafe. A suitably smug Richard Granger, head of the much derided Connecting for Health (CfH) programme, claimed if he'd been in charge of MTAS, such a breach would not have occurred. Channel 4 then discovered that the personal details (private addresses, phone numbers, e-mails, mobiles) of doctors attending a CfH conference were left up on its website for two weeks after the breach was reported and could still be obtained by Google-whack months later.

Hurrah for Heart Surgeons

On a brighter note, heart surgeons have shown the benefits of publishing sensitive data. Public disclosure of death rates began in 2001, after the Kennedy report on the deaths of child heart patients in Bristol. The death rate for coronary artery bypass graft (CABG) patients after public disclosure was significantly lower than it had been before, falling from 2.4% to 1.8% with no evidence that higher-risk patients were denied surgery.[1] The difference here is that grass-roots doctors are collecting data

[1] Bridgewater et al. Has the publication of cardiac surgery outcome data been associated with changes in practice in Northwest England? *Heart* Jan. 2007; doi:10.1136/hrt.2006.106393

and sharing it with patients because they believe it to be the right thing to do. Whereas Connecting for Health, Modernising Medical Careers and much of the Blair health reforms are ill-conceived, rushed, top-down disasters that are forced on the front line without consultation or agreement. They funnel billions away from patients into the pockets of private companies and they don't work. Blair may claim after ten years that he's saved the NHS, but he won't be around on August 1 when those juniors who haven't given up are still scrabbling around for jobs, and patients are wondering if they'll ever see a doctor.

What Should Gordon Do?

15 June 2007
What should Gordon Brown do with the NHS? He may want to put his 'unique stamp' on it, but Blairites are working around the clock to progress the market reforms beyond the point of no return. The great con of Blair's NHS was to preach the rhetoric of patient power whilst handing over control, and a vast sum of public money, to the private sector. To argue that this is not privatisation of the NHS is nonsense, but then Blair excelled at that.

The tipping point for the NHS will come if Labour pushes through its plans to outsource up to £64 billion worth of commissioning to multinational corporations such as United Health. This would suit Blair's friends at McKinsey, who can charge a fortune to the NHS for brokering the deals and also represent many of the US companies who stand to gain. At least one senior executive at McKinsey has a staff pass at the Department of Health. In return, Blair will have ample boot-filling opportunities in America.

In Blair's absence, Patsy Hewitt is rushing through his agenda before her exit, aided by David 'Nibbler' Nicholson, the surprise choice as NHS chief executive, who leapt up the shortlist after a meeting with Blairite health guru Professor Paul Corrigan. Nicholson in turn has appointed an NHS management team that is putting intense pressure on strategic health authorities and PCTs to outsource their commissioning. The idea that PCTs will retain ultimate control (and hence keep the NHS public) is a myth.

So what is Brown to do? Clearly a return to the Old Labour Stalinism of diktat by bureaucracy is impossible. And yet Blair's model is equally didactic, suggesting market competition is the only way forward and peppering it with promises of choice, when patients only get to choose what the Government (or United Health) wants them too. The junior doctor selection crisis is the most extreme example of this – thousands of doctors who have worked for seven years or more in the NHS are allowed only one choice of job, in many cases only specifying a region (e.g. Scotland) rather than a hospital unit. Stalin invented the internal market, the Tories introduced it to the NHS and Blair is polishing it to imperfection.

The NHS works because it is a one-stop shop – once you're in it, you get all the care you need. Contrast this to America, where patients who have brain tumours removed are sent home the next day if the insurance package does not include continuing care. If American managed-care corporations unleash their 'expertise' on the NHS, only an American system can result. Profitable patients are cherry-picked while unprofitable patients are dumped.

Brown must reverse this without seeming to be Old Labour. The solution is to deliver what Blair and Hewitt have pretended to promise: 'a devolved NHS where 80% of the decisions are made locally'. Working in the NHS is like pulling people out of a river without bothering to look at who's pushing them in. If Labour really wants patients to get involved in shaping services, it has to move the money upstream and stop the dysfunctional schism between top-down marketing and local decision-making. Most NHS resources now go on managing chronic illness, and many patients manage themselves perfectly well for all but three hours a year, when they're hanging round the surgery or outpatient clinic. Tapping into this expertise and getting patients to help other patients in their communities is the best hope of stopping the log-jam downstream. The message is simple. Local partnerships between patients and NHS staff work, market reforms don't. But will Brown swallow it?

ALAN JOHNSON
June 2007–

Alan 'Postie' Johnson might have anticipated an exciting new dawn under Gordon Brown, with perhaps even a pop at Prime Minister. Alas, he's now in Stephen Dorrell mode, overseeing the fag end of the 'new' Labour reform programme and trying to safe guard its legacy. He needn't worry too much. If you cut up the current Labour and Tory health plans (which is quite therapeutic in itself) and mix them up, it's very hard to tell them apart. The English NHS, at least, appears stuck with the market.

Johnson has been largely been outshone by Lord Darzi, a Labour peer who looks ideally placed to jump ship to the Tories, should the need arise. Darzi's review of the NHS echoed just about all of Frank Dobson's commitments to quality and safety, but the methods are very different. The ideological fault line between those who believe in competition as the best way to provide a health service, and those wedded to co-operation, is now so deep that it appears unbridgeable. The Department of Health is trying to come up with a third way – 'co-opetition' – but we've had our fill of 'new' Labour bullshit.

Labour still argues fervently that patients want choice, and I tend to agree. But only if the choice is based on meaningful and useful information. After eleven years of Labour, we still don't have accurate, comparative outcome data or defined safety standards to protect patients. Not all this is Labour's fault – quality and safety need to be grown from the bottom up, and it's up to NHS staff to lead the charge. But politicians have to embrace this focus on safety, not bury it under the guff of needless reform and secretive competition. Andrew Lansley take note.

PRIVATE EYE
Flash Darzi Saves the World

12 July 2007

New health secretary Alan Johnson's charm offensive on the NHS was delayed by the weather, but he seems to have cottoned on to the fact that you can't run an organisation of 1.3 million people from a box in Whitehall, part-time, while the great over-washed in Hull are demanding parity in flood defences with Sheffield.

So instead, it's up to junior heath minister Professor Ara Darzi, an Armenian born in Baghdad and trained in Ireland, to save the NHS part-time, in between minimally invasive robot-assisted surgery and a family. The Darzi review of the NHS in London lists a long line of previous reviews that made no difference to the vast inequalities in healthcare. But this time he's going to 'listen to Londoners, build a clinical consensus, provide evidence for the recommendations and work with the mayor and London boroughs'.

Alas, politicians need 'quick wins', which means not enough listening and too much change, too quickly. Johnson is already sounding quite the hypocrite, promising an end to top-down meddling in this new era of Brownian motion. Johnson also demonstrated his naivety by claiming the increase in life expectancy since the war was entirely due to the great scientific advances of the NHS, rather than largely due to economic and public health improvements.

Poor people get sick, and tackling poverty is a far better way of reducing health inequality than pouring money into the NHS. For those requiring NHS treatment, the biggest issue is the training and competence of the staff, rather than how healthcare is delivered (on the bus, in Tesco's, at a polyclinic). The front line of the NHS is very light on experience, and the generalists who can sort out the frail, obese elderly are a dying breed. Intensive care is full of 85-year-olds, slowly having the life sucked out of them and preventing further waiting-list reductions, and yet huge pressure is still piled on to hit the eighteen-week referral-to-treatment target. Less urgent patients leapfrog over the urgent every day. Johnson needs to give power for clinical decisions back to the staff, but will Brown be able to let go? Whatever happens, Darzi will survive. Anaesthetists often commit suicide because they have self-doubt and access to good drugs. Surgeons rarely do, because they are always right.

Child Ill-Health

20 August 2007

'There is now real concern and increasing evidence that the NHS is failing children.' So says Alan Craft, a professor of child health in Newcastle, in a *BMJ* editorial (August 11, 2007). This despite Labour's 'National Service Framework for Children', belatedly launched in 2004 in response to the Bristol scandal.

Alas, children don't vote and they tend not to take to the streets to complain about their care, so there was no additional money or specific targets for Labour's vision. Last year, the Healthcare Commission found that only 4% of trusts had made excellent progress in implementing the framework, and 21% rated good. Most progress was made in 'improving the hospital environment' but there was still 'a worrying potential for unsafe medical care'. That is, surgeons trained to operate on adults are still operating on children too, many on just a handful a year, making their results statistically meaningless.

Recruitment into high-risk, high-litigation paediatric specialties remains a problem and the service trundles on, with some hospitals lacking the staff to provide life support for children during the day and one in five unable to deal effectively with paediatric emergencies at night. The alternative, to close smaller units and merge services on fewer, bigger sites is politically unpalatable and they may still be unable to cope with the workload.

Good paediatric services are vital to the future of the NHS and without them the burden of chronic illness into adulthood is huge. The damage of passive smoking in pubs is negligible compared to the damage to a child if a mother smoked during pregnancy. If you survive your small, shrivelled placenta *in utero*, your risks of heart disease and premature death as an adult are greatly increased. I have written previously about the importance of fluoride for dental health, folic acid to prevent spina bifida and neonatal hearing tests to pick up deafness early, and yet the UK still has a lamentably poor record in preventative health for babies and children.

The UK also has one of the highest incidences of childhood diabetes and worst records of diabetic control, but the long-term devastation this causes is beyond the scope of short-term political targets. Our detection and survival rates for childhood cancer are amongst the worst in Europe and we're fifteenth in the European league table for perinatal mortality.

For the NHS to survive, it needs to invest in keeping children healthy upstream to prevent a log-jam later on. Programmes like SureStart and improvements in community child mental health services are starting to kick in but good hospital treatment is being stifled by targets for adult surgery and waiting times, and the difficulties in setting a fair tariff for complex paediatric care that requires input from many specialties. In a market NHS, paediatric care will only flourish if it can turn a profit. At present, much of it is cheap, unsafe and done on the hoof by non-specialists. Brown and Johnson need to refocus away from markets and back onto quality and safety.

Lord Darzi's Balls

4 October 2007

Who'd be Professor the Lord Darzi of Denham (FREng, KBE, FMedSci)? When asked by John Humphrys on the *Today* programme why his NHS review would be any different to any of the previous NHS reviews, he said 'Ee ah ah um colleagues.' He then trotted out the 'envy of the world' homily before being reminded that the NHS ranked seventeenth (out of 29) in the latest league table of European healthcare (behind Latvia). So should the NHS consider some level of charging? 'Governments will have to look at that in more clearly.' Eh?

No matter, there was still the hard copy of *Our NHS Our Future: NHS Next Stage Review Interim Report October 2007* to wade through. I hope this was rushed out as a cynical piece of electioneering. Otherwise, there's no excuse for 'we now need to change the way we lead change – effective change needs to be animated by the needs and preferences of patients, empowered to make their decisions count within the NHS with the response to patients' needs and choices being led by clinicians taking account of the best available evidence.'

I've never met a surgeon who speaks like that. Has Lord Darzi's brain been replaced with Labour arse gravy? 'Patients can feel like a number, rather than a person.' Hardly surprising when Choose and Book reduces you to a unique 12-digit PIN along with easy-to-remember computer-generated password ('fountain saver', 'broccoli spot', 'cake counter'). But the most striking claim is that the review 'is not about changing the way the NHS is structured'. So what is merging specialist services onto fewer sites, merging GPs into 'federated polyclinics' and downsizing district general hospitals?

Darzi has joined the party halfway through, when so much money has already been wasted on NHS change that he'll have a job convincing the staff of the need for more. He's proposing polyclinics to do much of the work done in district general hospitals, but we've already invested £1.4 billion in Independent Sector Treatment Centres that were supposed to do the same. ISTCs were encouraged into the market with guaranteed contracts paid above tariff. Last year, they were paid for 50,000 more operations than they carried out. The vast majority of waiting-list reductions were carried out in existing NHS hospitals and a huge sum has been wasted on unnecessary competition.

The NHS already has a competitive market under Payment By Results. Or rather activity. Hospitals can only survive by sucking as many patients as possible through their doors. ISTCs couldn't attract the custom, not least because they failed to submit sufficient outcome information to the Healthcare Commission to enable them to be audited for quality and safety.

Polyclinics may well have the expertise to treat patients closer to home but whether they can stand up to the might of desperate hospitals remains to be seen. To get the support of NHS staff, Darzi doesn't just need to consult them, he needs to publish evidence showing his reforms would work. The Academy of Medical Royal Colleges has performed the most comprehensive review of the reconfiguration plans and agrees that highly specialised services such as major trauma, heart and brain surgery need to be specialised on fewer sites. But it found no evidence to support the centralisation of the non-complex, high-volume work done in district general hospitals.

There is, however, evidence that patients feel access to GPs has improved in the last few years, which makes Brown and Darzi's peculiar focus on extending opening hours puzzling. The review smells strongly of hastily assembled populist opinion. Clinical medicine has been reformed in the last twenty years by focusing on the evidence, not the expert. The same needs to happen with NHS reform. Don't change the system until you can prove you've got something better.

Denying the Dying

14 November 2007

'What's the point of giving millions to cancer charities and spending billions on developing new drugs, often in the UK, if the NHS won't pay for them?' So asks Graham Smith, whose junior doctor son Ollie died from metastatic colon cancer at the age of 29, and who was denied the drug Avastin (bevacizumab) by Harrow PCT. The PCT was following guidance from NICE, which in January 2007 decided that Avastin did not represent a good enough use of NHS funds.

Strange, then, that it should be available across Europe and America. Avastin is a genetically engineered version of a mouse antibody that contains both human and mouse components. It is believed to work by inhibiting a protein that stimulates new blood vessels, thus denying tumors blood, oxygen and other nutrients needed for growth.

It is not a cure for metastatic cancer, but got its FDA licence in America in 2004 for use alongside chemotherapy because it 'has been proven to delay tumor growth and more importantly, significantly extend the lives of patients'. This may only be by a matter of months, but it can also extend the disease-free survival and so patients and relatives may be spared some of the relentless decline of metastatic cancer which transformed Ollie from 'a handsome fit young man to a grotesquely deformed blind and crippled old man in twelve weeks'.

Expensive as Avastin is (£2,500 per infusion), drug costs constitute a very small fraction of the overall cost to the NHS of treating cancer, with most resources spent in the last few months of life. If a drug keeps a patient out of hospital for longer, it could easily justify its cost. Roche, who manufacture the drug with Genentech, also make Herceptin and have a licence for Avastin in metastatic lung and breast cancer. Trials are ongoing to see if the drug works in early-stage cancers, where it has a better chance of cure, and the results are likely to lead to another lengthy bout of NICE deliberation. Roche has thus far played hardball with the price, arguing that it took over 30 years of research to find a monoclonal antibody able to delay tumour growth. They also believe the drug is worth the money, and that sufficient individuals and insurers will fork out, even if the NHS doesn't.

In May this year, the influential (and independent) Karolinska Institute in Sweden found that the 'excessive bureaucracy' involved in approving drugs for use (or not) in the NHS was one reason for our higher death rates. However, other European countries are looking at the NICE model as a way of containing their own drug costs and many also adopt its guidance.

All of which puts doctors in a difficult position. According to his father, Ollie's oncologist strongly recommended the use of Avastin in his treatment and thought the NHS would provide it. It was unanimously denied by the PCT initially and on appeal because of 'the duty to balance the needs of the individual with the needs of the wider population'. Had Ollie decided to take to the streets à la Herceptin ('young, handsome junior doctor who has given his life to caring for the sick denied vital cancer drug') he would doubtless have got it. Colon cancer in someone so young is rare, and its detection was doubtless delayed because of the long hours and hectic lifestyle of a trainee surgeon. Two doctors advised him he had irritable bowel syndrome.

Ollie's only demand was for his parents to reunite so he could die at home. His father remains incredulous that he was denied a licensed treatment, available in most other European countries. Living a few more months with a better quality of life doesn't sound like much until you try without.

Conflict of Interest: I have been paid to chair conferences for NICE and Roche. My views remain somewhere between the two.

In Praise of Bolton

1 February 2008

'By 2008, no-one will have to wait longer than eighteen weeks from GP referral to hospital treatment.' So said Labour's NHS Improvement Plan in June 2004. The definition of 'by 2008' is a little blurred. The key targets are that by March, 85% of patients needing hospital admission and 90% of those who don't should have a 'referral to treatment' time of eighteen weeks or less. It isn't until the end of December that it applies to all patients (but only if they want it to).

The 18-week website (www.18weeks.nhs.uk) has a helpful clock in the top left-hand corner (333 days to go!), but many PCTs are in despair about how to do it. 'Diagnostics' presents a particular challenge. When the target was announced, the waiting time in many areas for MRI scans was two years, but Bolton PCT has somehow managed to get the wait down for all diagnostic tests (apart from the odd six-week endoscopy) to two weeks.

So how's it done? Bolton PCT has some experienced, work-aholic and ballsy commissioners who were reasonably solvent when they started planning in 2005. Some of their solutions were obvious (getting Royal Bolton Hospital's imaging department to stay open over lunch), others were inspired (instead of pissing off all the consultants by parking a private scanner in the hospital car park, they took it into the community). They gave GPs direct access to urgent community scans for patients with abdominal pain and breathlessness, so they didn't have to be sent to A&E, kept in overnight and often not discharged for several days.

The growth of community scanning has forced the hospital to improve its service and the PCT can now insist that scans are reported on within four days (often sooner) with a treatment plan that the GP and patients can understand. And they're developing an IT system that allows the scans to be whizzed from hospital or scanner to GP surgery. By December 2007, 99% of patients who didn't need to be hospitalised were treated within eighteen weeks as were 92% of those who did.

Bolton is not the healthiest place to live – the life expectancy is several years less than, say, Dorset – but the fact that a deprived area has achieved such improvement when much of the rest of the NHS (particularly in the south) is still riven by petty, internecine, inter-professional rivalries is extraordinary.

Faster access to diagnostic tests is not a panacea. It's expensive, it encourages doctors to reach for the scanner rather than examine patients, it requires considerable operator skill, there is no mandatory regulation of the sonographers who perform ultrasounds, it throws up anxiety-provoking false results and it can increase exposure to unnecessary radiation. And under the old 'watch and wait' NHS rationing, some patients got better (or gave up) on their own. However, used correctly, a good scan will pick up your cancer, heart failure or leaking aneurysm far more quickly than if you sat at home waiting for the PCT and hospital to finish squabbling over who should be doing the scanning. So well done Bolton. Lord Darzi should pay them a visit.

Letter of the Week

15 February 2008

Sir,
I received Alan Johnson's letter today 'Improving access to GP services', and having just seen my last patient, I read it and thought I'd respond by phone. His number is on the letter. I spoke to a very nice chap and explained that having received Mr

Johnson's letter there were a couple of things I'd like to discuss with him. He asked me to hold and then came back on the line to say that Mr Johnson wasn't available, and in fact there was no one at all at the DoH who could discuss this letter with me, as they all go home by 5pm.

I'm delighted that at least everyone at the DoH finishes early enough to be able to see their own GP in a normal evening surgery without the need for extended opening hours.

Paul Baird

Portesham Surgery

Weymouth

The big fuss over extending GPs' hours has ended with Alan Johnson looking tough and the BMA looking foolish but the Government was never going to back down, knowing that GPs won't go on strike and precious few would abandon their NHS income and final salary pension scheme for the vicissitudes of private practice and the stock market. And given the current over-supply of doctors (6,000 new graduates each year but only 3,000 retiring), Labour knows that there is plenty of young blood desperate for work (one practice I work in had 70 applicants for a maternity locum). Alas, the proposed extension of hours has to come out of existing funds so most practices will just run a few nurse-led minor-illness clinics to mop up the commuters suffering First Great Western stress.

A bigger problem for Johnson (and patients) will be the longer-term damage caused by doctors' lack of engagement with his reforms. Hospitals had first shout at the 'constructive discomfort' of private competition to make them raise their game. Waiting lists came down and many of the Independent Sector Treatment Centre projects (having made a quick killing at the expense of the taxpayer) are now struggling for work, with new projects abandoned. The private sector sees general practice as a far more lucrative market – there are twelve million chronically sick patients out there likely to remain that way for life – but whether a United Health or Virgin polyclinic can provide the same service and value as traditional general practice remains to be seen. Doctors are competitive by nature and most will rise to the challenge, but their likelihood of succeeding is reduced by the unfair advantages ('incentives to enter the market') offered to the private sector. When Lord Darzi's GP adviser and Labour stalwart Sam Everington loses out to Atos Health in a bid to extend GP services in East London, most GPs will feel they haven't got a chance of beating the multinationals.

As for hospitals, foundation trusts are now free from Department of Health control and likely to concentrate on treatments that make money, rather than provide a comprehensive service for all patients. Unison has launched a judicial review against Monitor (the foundation-trust regulator) which currently allows the trusts to avoid a cap on private-patient income by setting up a separate company to provide treatment. So NHS hospitals are taking on private competition by privatising themselves. Such an aggressive, market-based system works beautifully in America.

Patient McChoice

21 March 2008

'The Good Hospital Guide. From Cardio to Cancer – where to get the best treatment.' So proclaims the front page of the *Independent* (March 20), to coincide with Labour's April 1 pledge that patients requiring non-emergency treatment can travel to any NHS hospital in England, or indeed any private one that has an NHS contract. Alas, the *Indy*'s extensive guide lists just ten 'best' hospitals, all in London. For 'eyes' it recommends Moorfields Hospital, whose latest Healthcare Commission rating for quality of services was 'weak', and for 'bones and joints' it goes for the Royal National Orthopaedic Hospital in Stanmore (HC rating, 'fair'). The Royal Marsden Hospital for cancer does at least have an 'excellent' rating but 'cancer is one of the specialties excluded from the extended patient choice agenda.'

The *Indy*'s sparse recommendations are entirely based on reputation, but patient choice is pointless without outcome data that provides a meaningful comparison between different centres for each specific treatment. How likely is it that the treatment will improve my quality of life? How likely is it that it will kill or maim me? The Government and NHS have been painfully slow to roll this information out for other specialties, but BUPA has been collecting patient-reported outcome measures (PROMs) since 1999, in the wake of the carnage caused by rogue gynaecologist Rodney 'the butcher' Ledward. Patients complete a standardised questionnaire (e.g. EQ–5D available at www.euroqol.org) and are followed up at three and six months after surgery. Prospective patients can then be given a fair indication of how likely a treatment is to improve quality of life rather than just providing a pathology specimen and a six-inch scar.

The NHS is only now dabbling with PROMs, limiting them to hernias, varicose veins and hip and knee replacements for 2008–09. This is a tacit acceptance that information gathering for BUPA (with largely middle-class, articulate, motivated patients) may be easier than following up NHS patients. A 70% response rate will require a huge amount of effort and my guess is that it will be dumped on GPs, who will refuse to do it.

In the meantime, patient choice will continue to be cosmetic and insubstantial. Hospitals can take on the most inappropriate corporate sponsors (some, such as Guy's, have had a McDonalds on site for years) and use their expertise to advertise services (but not directly discredit the services of their rivals). They can also enlist the help of celebrities who've been patients to publicly endorse the treatment they've received. Those who don't already jump the queue for a private room will be able to enhance their treatment with the promise of a free plug.

Most patients will choose to stick with their nearest hospitals but choice has the potential to improve quality and safety in the NHS by putting reliable, independent, unbiased performance data in the public domain and making all hospitals up their game. In contrast, adverts, sponsorship and celebrity endorsement will just be a breeding ground for yet more bias and spin.

The Politics of Prostate Cancer

10 April 2008

Why are men with early prostate cancer still being denied NICE-approved treatment? The disease kills ten thousand men a year, but the cancer is difficult to predict. In some it spreads rapidly and often presents too late for a cure, in others it remains localised in the prostate gland without causing any obvious harm. For the latter, radical surgery or radiotherapy may do more harm than good.

The research challenge is to develop better screening tests and identify those early cancers that are likely to spread. More localised treatments, which eradicate the cancer while sparing patients the misery of incontinence and impotence, are also needed. Brachytherapy, which inserts radioactive seeds into the prostate, is one such treatment for early cancer, and achieves as good a control of the disease as radical surgery with far fewer side-effects. Indeed, it is the only minimally invasive treatment for the disease that is approved by NICE (February 2008).

This should, in theory, give a much better choice for men who decide they want to be tested for the disease and are found to have localised cancer. They can either choose to have surveillance rather than treatment, with the option of doing something later if the cancer starts to grow (NICE's preferred and cheapest option). Or they can choose to go straight for treatment, preferably with the fewest side-effects. Brachytherapy became available in the UK a decade ago, but many patients have been denied funding for it on the NHS. There was a blanket ban on all new NHS referrals from Wales between October 2005 and February 2007, and men are still being denied treatment despite NICE approval.

Others have taken on their PCT and won. Roy Stainton is a retired professor of operational mathematics who was found to have localised prostate cancer in 2004. His consultant at Winchester Hospital gave him a 'prostate cancer treatment toolkit' to mull over, but tried to remove the section on brachytherapy because 'the PCT will never fund it.' Mr Stainton decided he wanted it and was swiftly declined.

Appealing against South Hants PCT wasn't easy. His GP knew very little about brachytherapy and he was left alone to assemble his case. He read up on the research, used it to inform his case, gathered letters of support and lodged his appeal. He was offered a hearing and the chance to respond to contrary evidence by the end of the day on which the letter arrived. He quickly reviewed the evidence and delivered his response by hand. He was also invited to take a medical representative with him, which he didn't have, and although the nice lady from the Patient Advocacy Liaison Service was keen, she didn't know anything about brachytherapy either.

At the hearing, the PCT mislaid his supplementary evidence, which was subsequently photocopied and circulated. Mr Stainton's statistical analysis showed that, when all convalescence costs were considered, brachytherapy was no more expensive than radical surgery, and cheaper in the long term if side-effects were avoided. Labour would no doubt claim this was patient advocacy in action. In reality, you're on your own and it helps if you're a statistical genius.

For every successful appeal, there are many more losers. Men are remortgaging their houses and going to small private clinics rather than larger specialist centres with the expertise to do brachytherapy properly.[1] The NICE guidance should finally end this, and make high-quality treatment available to all who choose it, but don't hold your breath.

[1] http://www.prostatebrachytherapyinfo.net/

Bring Back Safety First

8 May 2008

'I want to help use Elaine's death to help bring cultural change in healthcare. I want to tell our two young children when they have grown up that Mummy's death has made a big difference.' So says inspirational pilot Martin Bromiley on the website for his charity founded to recognise the role of human factors in the prevention of medical error (www.chfg.org).

Elaine Bromiley was 37 and healthy when she was booked in for non-emergency sinus surgery under general anaesthesia in a private unit adjacent to an NHS hospital. Her consultant anaesthetist had sixteen years of experience, the ENT surgeon had 30 years under his belt, and three of the four nurses in the theatre were also very experienced. The theatre was very well equipped, there were no competing pressures of emergencies elsewhere, but there was another senior anaesthetist operating in the theatre next door. As Bromiley observed: 'This was a dream scenario for safety. A senior, competent surgical team working in state-of-the-art surroundings.'

Anaesthesia was induced at 08.35 but it was not possible to insert the laryngeal mask airway. By 08.37, oxygenation began to deteriorate and she looked cyanosed. Her oxygen saturation dropped to 75% (anything below 90% is significantly low). By 08.39 oxygen saturation had fallen to 40% but attempts to ventilate the lungs with 100% oxygen using a facemask and oral airway proved extremely difficult. The saturation level remained perilously low but the anaesthetist, who was joined by a consultant colleague, was unable to perform a tracheal intubation.

By 08.45, airway access had still not been achieved and the situation was termed 'can't intubate, can't ventilate', a recognised emergency for which guidelines (requiring an emergency tracheotomy to establish an airway through the front of the neck) were well known. One nurse, on her own initiative, fetched the tracheotomy tray. Another, recognising the severity of the situation, went to secure a bed on the intensive care unit. However, the three consultants decided to keep attempting intubation, unsuccessfully, and at 09.10 abandoned the procedure hoping she would wake up. Her oxygen saturation had remained at less than 40% for twenty minutes and she never recovered consciousness, dying thirteen days later.

Martin Bromiley was initially told that his wife's death was extreme bad luck and that nothing more could have been done. As a pilot, he was used to analysing critical incidents in a no-blame culture and wanted to hear the results of the ensuing inquiry. He was told: 'There won't be an inquiry. Not unless you complain or sue.' Bromiley insisted on an independent expert review, which concluded that, given the skill mix of the clinicians, it should have been very easy to follow the established emergency protocol and perform a tracheotomy. So why didn't it happen?

Errors in medicine happen not just because of lack of skill or knowledge but for behavioural reasons. Ask doctors what they should do in an exam, and they trot out the guidelines. Put them in the extremely stressful situation of a very rare, rapidly deteriorating potential catastrophe and even the most senior clinicians can lose the plot. The role of these human factors in decision-making is well recognised in aviation and it is to his enormous credit that Bromiley has assembled leaders in the field to work out how such disasters can be prevented. Simulating emergency situations, pre-briefing and debriefing before surgery, introducing and valuing members of the team and creating a culture where the most junior member of staff (or even the patient) can raise concerns or call for a time-out sound obvious, but don't happen routinely in the NHS. And the drive for productivity and cost-containment under Labour is leading to yet more corner-cutting. For the sake of Elaine Bromiley, and the thousands of others who die each year from avoidable error, Lord Darzi's review must rebuild the NHS around safety.

Why Children Still Die

6 June 2008
Why Children Die, a detailed analysis of UK childhood death in 2006 (and published last month), has concluded that in 69% of deaths, there were avoidable or potentially avoidable factors. Equally alarming for a report that should be central to the reform of the NHS is that it has received virtually no publicity.

In the study, carried out by the Confidential Enquiry into Maternal and Child Health (CEMACH) with funding from the National Patient Safety Agency (NPSA), data was gathered on 957 deaths of children in three English regions, Wales and Northern Ireland. An expert panel examined 119 deaths in detail but the 'headline result of the panel data' is hidden away on page 47. According to one panel member, the release of the report was delayed by Labour citing purdah and neutered in response to pressure from the Cabinet Office and the Department of Health.

So what has the Government got to be frightened of? Despite a succession of declarations on patient safety, such as *An Organisation with a Memory*, and a large safety conference attended by Gordon Brown last month, the NHS appears not to be learning much from either the Bristol or Climbie disasters. In both medical and social care, children are still not getting access to expertise quickly enough. The recurring patterns of substandard care are depressingly familiar: poor care of sick children by staff not adequately trained in paediatrics or supervised by those who are; failure to recognise a sick/vulnerable child; failure of follow-up; failure to immunise; failure to refer to mental health services. Some of the findings were unexpected (e.g. high rates of child suicide), but avoidable factors related to clinical and organisational care were far more predictable and possibly made worse by the Government's reforms.

The devolution of frontline NHS care to the least experienced (and cheapest) staff is commonplace and 'in 8% of hospital trusts, surgeons carrying out elective surgery did not perform enough work with children to maintain their skills.' So why are strategic health authorities, commissioners and trusts allowing them to do it? Because trusts need the money and no-one is brave enough to enforce safety standards. And the current obsession with public involvement is cementing the future of small, inadequately staffed paediatric units serving similar maternity units. The public (and politicians) love a cosy local unit but no-one has the balls to tell them that lives are at risk when emergencies are badly managed.

The obsession with performance targets has meant many children have been erased from outpatient clinics if they fail to attend but trusts are making no attempt to detect those most at risk (who are hardly to blame if an adult forgets or isn't able to take them to hospital). Many operational policies and pathways still don't reflect best practice, referrals to the Coroner's office are still not managed properly and death certificates are still littered with errors.

On a brighter note, there were plenty of examples of excellent practice but, as ever, the NHS hopes that good care will spread by some mysterious osmosis from beacon sites rather than building reform from the bottom up on quality and safety. As of April, Local Safeguarding Children Boards have been set up to continue studying child deaths, but their current methodology (looking at unexpected deaths) will not identify all avoidable factors outlined in this excellent CEMACH study. There are salutary lessons here for everyone who works in (and uses) the NHS, but the fact that I only heard of *Why Children Die* from a concerned *Eye* reader reveals how far Labour has to go before being open about the true extent of medical error.

The Ben Bradshaw Fan Club

17 June 2008

'Dear Ben Bradshaw. Regarding your recent comments about the BMA Save Our Surgery campaign having a "misleading and mendacious nature". Fuck off, you ugly, duplicitous cunt.'

This top-quality posting (373 votes and counting) on June 12 from a London trainee surgeon, appeared on the 'Air Your Views to the Media' forum of Doctors.net.uk, 'the largest professional forum of UK doctors.'[1] Other doctors quickly weighed in with their views on the health minister: 'Floppy-haired cuntistic fuckwit' (from a consultant psychiatrist), 'liar', 'ignorant pain in the arse' and 'odious little creep' (from three

---

[1] *Why Children Die.* CEMACH 2008. ISBN 978-0-9558055-0-9.

GPs). Bradshaw, who sees himself as a mini-Milburn enforcer, would doubtless be delighted with the feedback. But why do doctors dislike him so much?

Bradshaw was wheeled out to defuse the BMA's petition of 1.2 million patient signatures, gathered in just three weeks, opposing polyclinic plans that threaten thousands of GP surgeries. Bradshaw was unimpressed: 'I am not surprised the BMA have collected so many signatures given the misleading and mendacious nature of their campaign. If I were to run a campaign making false claims that something terrible was about to happen, a lot of people would sign my petition too.'

So after eleven years of Labour and a year of Lord Darzi running around the UK trying to engage and inspire NHS staff, politicians and doctors still hate each other. With such a dysfunctional relationship at the centre of the NHS, it's no wonder the UK still has such poor health outcomes.

General practice certainly needs some help – some deprived areas are very under-doctored and the quality of service is distinctly variable. Most doctors (and many patients) would rather the Government invested in and expanded existing services rather than introduce large, often privately owned, health centres, but Labour is determined to have some more shiny buildings to show off come election time, never mind the quality.

Labour's claims that having a polyclinic on your doorstep will not affect the viability of existing GP practices is clearly nonsense. As with Independent Sector Treatment Centres, the private sector is very good at creaming off 'easy' patients and leaving the NHS to pick up all the difficult ones. With a recession looming, money is tight enough in the NHS without splashing out on 150 new clinics. And polyclinics can only be staffed by importing experienced doctors from abroad, poaching them from neighbouring practices, or filling them with newly qualified GPs with no senior support to hand.

Continuity and teamwork are central to general practice. Patients, particularly those with chronic illnesses, value relationships built up over time and there's a limit to what you can achieve in six minutes with a stranger. Even more problematic for Labour's plans is Lord Darzi's assertion that all reform must be based on evidence, and evidence for the value of polyclinics over traditional general practice does not exist, according to the King's Fund.

Some GP practices have relocated to larger centres and are delivering excellent, expanded services, but the move was their decision and they have ensured that continuity and teamwork have not been disrupted. But most GPs are sitting tight and ignoring Labour. As one put it: 'There's no point engaging with the fag end of a government. Soon the Tories will be in, they'll reintroduce fundholding and we'll be back where we started in 1997.' Ah, the smell of progress.

Darzi's Déjà Vu Review

1 July 2008
Will Lord Darzi be following Raj Persaud to the GMC on charges of plagiarism? His NHS review, *High Quality Care For All* (June 30, 2008), is alarmingly similar to Frank Dobson's 1998 bestseller, *A First Class Service: Quality in the New NHS*. Dobson's foreword starts: 'All patients in the National Health Service are entitled to high quality care', and promises that 'unacceptable variations that have grown up in recent years must end.' Just ten years later, Darzi stresses that tackling significant variations in the quality of care will be his first priority.

Dobson's reforms would ensure 'high quality care becomes the norm everywhere.' Darzi, in contrast, will deliver 'high quality for users of services in all aspects, not just some'. Dobson manages 191 mentions of 'quality' in his document compared to Darzi's 359. But Dobson put quality in every chapter heading (Setting Quality Standards, Delivering Quality Standards, Monitoring Quality Standards and Action for Quality.) So the claim that the Darzi review is radically different for its focus on quality is clearly bollocks.

Dobson put his paper out for consultation but Darzi has already consulted over 2,000 doctors and the fact that so many put variation in quality at the top of their agenda a decade after Labour promised to abolish it is frankly disturbing. In his foreword, Brown desperately tries to rewrite history by claiming that the first ten years of Labour were all about building capacity to get waiting lists down, and now it's time to focus on, um, quality. Perhaps he was sulking when Dobson tried just that.

There are lots of other similarities – promises to put patients at the centre of care, gather their opinions and give them outcome figures – but two key differences. Dobson's log made not a single mention of the word 'choice'. Darzi gives us 62 to choose from. Dobson is Old Labour, believes in co-operation in healthcare (along with the Scottish and Welsh assemblies) and that people don't want to shop around for treatment when they're ill. Blair quickly got rid of him and brought in Milburn to feed the NHS to the market. Lots of money, duplication and job insecurity has indeed got waiting lists down, but because the publication of clinical outcomes promised by Dobson and Milburn has never materialised, we still don't know if the onslaught on waiting lists will come at the price of failed cataract surgery and joint replacements later on. Quicker does not always mean better.

Dobson also believed that the healthy competition of professionalism would raise standards but Darzi has swallowed the Blair belief that staff need financial incentives to practise good care. So as well as reminding them to treat patients with dignity and respect (doh!), they will be paid extra for providing a 'new' quality service based on outcomes. Could this be an extension of the quality and outcomes framework that 'incentivised' GPs so well? Incentives work by undermining the neutrality of professional judgement and encouraging self-interested decision-making. They wouldn't be needed if good information on outcomes was published.

So, has the fag end of Labour got the stomach to do what it promised a decade ago? I first called for heart surgeons to publish their results back in 1992 and now they are doing so, but no-one else is. In 2001, the Paediatric Cardiac Services Review that followed the Kennedy inquiry recommended the number of units performing child heart surgery be reduced from thirteen to six to ensure quality and safety. There are still thirteen, because putting babies at risk is trumped by the political risk of closing a local service. On July 18, 2001, Alan Milburn promised in the Commons he would publish 'information for patients, and specifically for parents, before consenting to treatment for themselves or their children'. To date it has not appeared. If the last 60 years has taught us anything about the NHS, it's that – Nye Bevan aside – politicians can't deliver the hard stuff. Don't give up the day job, Darzi.

Not Warts and All

16 July 2008

Why has Labour chosen not to protect girls from genital warts as well as cervical cancer? I have written previously about the UK's delay in instigating a vaccination programme with Gardasil, which gives excellent protection against both diseases and has been widely used for over a year in the US, Canada, Australia and many European countries. Not only has the UK delayed introduction – presumably for cost reasons – but it has plumped for a cheaper vaccine, Cervarix, which only protects against cervical cancer.

Those unsure of how unpleasant warts can be should take a peek at http://www.chestersexualhealth.co.uk/genitalwarts.htm. Be warned – it isn't for the squeamish. I've worked in a sexual clinic and seen the devastation that warts cause to people's sex lives (often non-existent) and emotional well-being (sometimes profoundly depressed). They're extremely common, with upwards of 85,000 cases a year in England and Wales, costing £25 million annually to treat. There would have been a significant reduction in wart workload and anguish within a few years had Gardasil been chosen, and in time, the savings would easily compensate for the disparity in price between the two vaccines.

Labour's decision makes no economic, clinical or humane sense. On January 16, a letter from health secretary Alan Johnson to Colm O'Mahony, a sexual health consultant, suggests that Labour were at that stage opting for Gardasil: 'It is expected the vaccination of girls will reduce the transmission of infection to boys, by herd immunity, and reduce the number of genital warts cases in boys as well as girls.' So why the change of mind? Labour spouts all this guff about respecting and understanding patients and then makes an absurdly unempathic decision.

Johnson's prevarication over top-up payments centres on his dislike of two-tier health systems, but every sexual health consultant and GP I've spoken to is advising parents who can afford it to pay for Gardasil (£250 for three injections). Why would you not protect your daughter against warts if you could? Some doctors have had their sons vaccinated too. Warts can kill your sex life, treatment can be embarrassing and uncomfortable, and in a third of people they keep coming back.

Perhaps the market reforms of the NHS have left it so bankrupt that there simply isn't enough spare cash to fund the more expensive vaccine. But given that foundation hospitals have made record savings and are sitting on over £1 billion of taxpayers' money, this doesn't stack up. Labour – 'the champions of choice' – are denying parents the right to choose whether to protect their daughters against what can be a psychologically devastating, chronic infection. At the very least, those parents whose daughters are due to join the cervical cancer vaccination programme and want them to have the extra protection should be allowed to pay the difference between the two vaccines, rather than pay the whole cost of Gardasil. This is one top-up that's worth it.

Market Balls

1 August 2008

The key to the success of Lord Darzi's next-stage review is to 'put clinicians back in the driving seat' of the NHS. But do they understand where they're going? The service is now riddled with jargon invented by management consultants to justify their fee, and very few doctors have a clue what it means. Additionality. Contestibility. Service Line Reporting. Patient Level Activity Based Costing Solutions. Directed Enhanced Services. Extended Choice Network. Healthcare Resource Group version 4. Market Forces Factor. Secondary Users' Services. Unbundling the Tariff.

The situation is so dire that this year's Audit and Healthcare Commission report on Labour's reforms, *Is the Treatment Working?*, had to include a five-page glossary. Unsurprisingly, the report concluded there is no evidence that the imposition of choice and competition is improving the service. The Healthcare Commission's reward is to disappear up the arse of the new Quality Care Commission, where it will find it much harder to cause trouble.

According to the *Health Service Journal* (July 24), GPs keen on getting involved in practice-based commissioning (whatever that is) are not communicating well with PCTs when submitting 'service redesign bids'. So to help them write their business plans, everyone's favourite health minister Ben Bradshaw is bringing in more management consultants 'to establish a framework contract providing quality assured development support'.

Occasionally, doctors understand only too well what managers are getting at. The *HSJ* also reported a 'brutal culling' at Avon and Wiltshire Mental Health Trust, which has decided to replace its medical director (i.e. a doctor trying her hand at management), along with the finance director, while asking four other managers to reapply for their roles. I have now been sent the eight-page advert for the new combined role of medical director and director of strategy and business development.

The trust is looking for a doctor to 'drive the business development strategy in line with the Business Proposition, scanning the mental health environment for new opportunities and identifying and stimulating new business solutions that fit with the corporate vision'. The ad mentions 'profitability' four times. We no longer treat the mentally ill according to need. We have to make money out of them.

I have also been sent a draft contract between Dr Foster Research, the private company making millions out of (our) NHS data and drug-giant Pfizer. The contract is for a 'customised version of the population health manager tool' for £375,000 plus VAT. The tool uses NHS data to allow analysis of 'market sizing, hospital market share, GP referral patterns, benchmarking provider performance and understanding admission rates'. This will allow Pfizer to 'focus marketing and awareness-raising activity to stimulate growth'.

Labour's reforms can't succeed because, despite all Darzi's rhetoric of 'engagement', you can only unite the NHS around common values, and the emphasis on commodity and profitability is repugnant to many frontline staff. Labour can try to disguise its agenda through the bullshit of marketisation, but it still smells terrible.

Letter for Publication

11 August 2008

> *Fundamentals and the new Quality Care Commission (sic)*
>
> Glad to see the *Eye* tradition of getting names wrong still flourishes. We are the Care Quality Commission. The Healthcare Commission won't disappear up our fundament but will be embraced by the new Care Quality Commission and we will carry forward proudly its values of independent and tough evidence and information on the quality of health and social care. Fundamental!
>
> Yours sincerely,
> Barbara Young
> Chair
> Care Quality Commission

Pass the Buck

15 August 2008

Labour made a big issue of publishing hospital-specific survival rates for three operations last month on the NHS Choices website (www.nhs.uk) But much of the information has mysteriously disappeared and no guidance is available for any of my local hospitals other than 'the survival rate is within the expected range'.

When the figures were initially released (and published in the *Guardian*, July 7, 2008), NHS director Bruce Keogh assured us that 'no hospital was unsafe' despite some hospitals having nearly four times the expected mortality rates for repair of abdominal aortic aneurysms (AAA, a potentially fatal ballooning of the main blood vessel).

Quite how this equates with safety is unclear. As data is collated from different hospitals, a 'statistical outlier detection system' should pick up units which are a long way below average. This should then prompt a swift investigation to ascertain whether this is down to bad luck (e.g. a run of deaths occurring by chance together in an otherwise good set of results) or because a surgical team takes on harder operations in sicker patients. Or is it because the team has gone off the boil or is struggling to learn a new technique? Most pertinently, does surgery need to be suspended pending a fuller investigation to protect patients?

This level of scrutiny appears beyond the Department of Health, despite a paper in the *British Journal of Surgery* from St George's Hospital which found that there are indeed significant outliers in the UK for AAA repair. But the DoH has never been keen on 'getting involved in clinical matters'. As far back as 1989, the Bristol unit (now one of the best in the UK) was identified as a significant outlier for paediatric cardiac surgery but was allowed to struggle on until 1995, when as many as 35 babies under one year old died unnecessarily.

This information was hidden from the public but the latest approach seems to be to publish it (if only momentarily) and then let patients choose whether they'd like to go to their nearest trust with cheap parking, nice coffee and four times the mortality rate. Or make a long trip to a strange hospital with a better survival rate (parking permitting).

The Royal Colleges are supposed to set statistical standards in medicine and surgery but, like the Department of Health, they have generally shied away for fear that someone high-profile and litigious (perhaps even a senior member of the college) might fall short. But passing the buck to patients to choose what mortality rates they're prepared to accept without any attempt to rein in hospitals that are way off the scale is a dereliction of duty.

Collecting outcomes is clearly a good thing, but they need

intelligent statistical analysis and action against units that are a long way behind the pack. You can't just say all units are 'safe' without a statistical definition of what safety means. Statistics don't provide all the answers, particularly if a unit does so few of an operation that the figures are meaningless. Complex surgery should be concentrated in units that have the resources and expertise to do lots of operations and prove they can do them well. But instead of stopping dabblers from operating, the Department of Health is just publishing their figures and hoping either that patients won't choose to go there, or that surgeons will choose not to do occasional operations, knowing that one death will send them plummeting to the bottom of the league. Labour doesn't want to be seen to be the one to close a local unit if the figures aren't up to scratch, because closure of anything always loses votes. So it's all down to patient choice (if the figures reappear).

Dangerous Surgery (No. 467)

29 August 2008

What's the definition of dangerous surgery? When you do the wrong thing (turn up pissed, cut off the wrong leg), it's obvious. But what if a surgical team attempts the correct procedure, but the patients keep dying? If you analyse each unexpected death (which doesn't always happen), you may spot something in the process of the operation (e.g. the surgeon was very slow) that might identify the problem. But for major surgery, a certain number of patients will die even in the best hands, and often it will take a number of operations for a pattern to emerge. Here, you need a statistical definition of danger to tell you that you are significantly worse at a particular operation than the average surgical team in the NHS, and you should stop operating and investigate.

That's the theory, but sixteen years after the *Eye* exposed the comparatively dangerous results for complex child heart surgery in Bristol, neither the Department of Health nor the Royal College of Surgeons has introduced such a statistical benchmark and, as a result, dangerous surgery still flourishes in the NHS. The General Medical Council covered its arse in 1998 by disciplining the Bristol surgeons for failing to act on their poor results, but the judgement was nonsensical without a statistical definition of poor. Without such a benchmark, you don't know when to stop.

The subsequent Public Inquiry nearly got there by spotting that a baby's overall chance of dying after complex heart surgery in Bristol between 1991 and 1995 was double the average rate in all the other NHS units. 'Double-the-average-mortality-elsewhere' should have been adopted as the danger benchmark across a whole range of major surgery where death is a significant risk. It would also require a surgical unit to prove its safety by doing enough of a particular operation to provide statistically significant results, and to carefully code and count each procedure to ensure the data was accurate.

Researchers at St George's Hospital in London have used this standard to analyse the repair of abdominal aortic aneurysms (AAA) in England between 2001 and 2005.[1] Hospitals which had a statistically significant mortality rate more than twice the average in the rest of the English NHS were identified as dangerous. The average mortality rate was 7.4%. Three English hospitals had mortality rates above 14.8% and 30 had rates consistently greater than 7.4%. Units needed to be performing at least 32 operations a year to produce statistically meaningful results, and the units performing the most operations generally

[1] Demonstrating safety through in-hospital mortality analysis. *British Journal of Surgery* 2008; 95: 64–71.

got better results. A similar (unpublished) analysis up to March 31, 2007, has again identified three dangerous units.

So why has Bruce Keogh, clinical director of the NHS, said that no unit performing AAA repair is unsafe, despite his own figures showing units with nearly four times the average mortality rate? Why did Lord Darzi, a surgeon himself, not define a statistical safe standard in his tortuous review? And why isn't Barbara Young, *Eye*-reading chair of the new Care Quality Commission, stopping units that can't prove their safety and investigating those where there is proof that they are dangerous? Similar statistical outliers exist for other operations, such as carotid endarterectomy and angioplasty. One lesson from Bristol is that if you collect outcomes, but don't act on the results, you're courting disaster. In the meantime, all patients wanting safe surgery should ask: 'Do you do enough of these procedures to produce statistically meaningful results?' and if so, 'Is your death rate more than double the average elsewhere in the NHS?' Then you have a choice . . .

Letter to Barbara Young, Chair, Care Quality Commission

29 August 2008

Dear Barbara
Thank you for your letter to *Private Eye* pointing out my error. One of the strengths of the *Eye* is that it's very good at admitting to and publishing mistakes. Far better, I would suggest, than the NHS. I trust you felt your correction was given due prominence.

I wonder if, in return, you could do something

for me? For the last sixteen years, I have exposed a succession of dangerous surgery scandals in the *Eye*. They will shortly be published together in a book, along with this letter, and I will send you a copy. Several themes emerge, which are summarised in the attached *Eye* column, and which I think the Care Quality Commission should urgently address.

We need to stop surgical units from performing complex surgery occasionally because, irrespective of the outcome, the results are always statistically meaningless and so such units can never provide proof of their safety to patients. This necessarily involves the reconfiguration and centralisation of some services which Labour has promised for many years, but not achieved.

To do this, we need to use the most accurate and up-to-date NHS data we have to calculate the minimum annual caseload of procedures that will achieve statistical significance. For example, researchers at St George's Hospital in London have concluded that for non-urgent Abdominal Aortic Aneurysm repair, it is 32.

We then need to set a statistical safety standard that is meaningful to patients and will identify potentially dangerous units. A mortality rate of more than double the average rate in all the other NHS units seems a good benchmark to me.

By this standard, the St George's research team has identified three dangerous units for AAA repair in England, which I think you should investigate. The Vascular Society knows where they are, and I'm sure they could assist you in this matter. Bruce Keogh has said that no AAA unit is unsafe, but hasn't defined safety and his recent analysis found that some units have more than three times the expected mortality rate. I just don't understand this.

It would be reassuring to know that, in its 60th year, the NHS might finally do something meaningful to protect patients from unsafe surgery. By the 'double-the-average-death-rate-elsewhere' criterion, there is still a lot of dangerous surgery in the NHS, and even more with no evidence of safety. As with Bristol, everyone in authority is aware of this problem, but no-one has the balls to address it. I'm hoping you're that person. Please let me know how you get on.

Yours sincerely,

Dr Phil Hammond (MD, *Private Eye*)

Cc Bruce Keogh, Clinical Director, Department of Health

Ara Darzi, Health Minister

Graeme Catto, President, General Medical Council

E-mail from Sir Graeme Catto, President, General Medical Council

Sent: Sun 31/08/2008 20:06

Phil

Thanks – I'll discuss this with my colleagues and get back to you whenever possible.

Graeme

E-mail from Lord Darzi, health minister

Sent: Mon 01/09/2008 00:07
Dear Phil,
Thank you for the email. I will ask the DH to respond to this if Bruce has not already.
Best wishes
Ara

Letter from Barbara Young, Chair, Care Quality Commission

9, September, 2008

Dear Dr Hammond,
Thank you for your letter of 29th August about investigations into surgical safety, and for the advance copy (and advance warning) of your *Private Eye* column published last week. The Care Quality Commission exists currently in shadow form only and has very few staff who could consider these issues. It will not commence its functions formally until April next year and therefore has no regulatory or investigatory powers until then.

The issues you raised in your letter and column are currently the responsibility of the Healthcare Commission. I have therefore passed your query on to Anna Walker, who will respond more fully to your points shortly.

Yours sincerely,
Barbara Young

To Be Continued (if anyone can be arsed to set safety standards for surgery). Meanwhile, back in GP-land . . .

Danger! GPs at work

11 September 2008

How safe is general practice? No-one really knows, because no-one collects any data. The National Patient Safety Agency has a National Reporting and Learning System (NRLS) for near misses and cock-ups anywhere in the NHS. It's confidential and voluntary, supposedly to encourage participation. Of the 80,000 reports it receives each month, 5% come from community pharmacies and 1% from GPs. Considering 90% of healthcare occurs outside hospitals, it's a piss-poor effort.

There is good evidence from the airline industry, and increasingly from hospitals, that the more errors you report, the less likely you are to harm people. This seems counter-intuitive but organisations that collect, analyse and learn from minor errors are far better at preventing serious ones. Many GP practices have audit meetings behind closed doors, where they discuss complaints, deaths and any bodge-ups that may have been spotted. This is generally done in a supportive, no-blame manner, even when there's clear evidence that someone has made a rudimentary error. And the error is hardly ever reported, least of all by a GP. Most of the NRLS reports from primary care are about vaccination, suggesting they come from nurses.

All clinical staff make mistakes and the error count is rising as medicine becomes more complex. But without a systematic way of picking up and learning from errors, it's likely that the same ones just keep repeating themselves. Recently, I attended a Medicine Safety in Practice conference in Manchester which discussed prescribing errors so serious that they couldn't be hidden. The first concerned a man on long-term warfarin therapy to reduce his risk of a stroke. He also suffered from arthritis. Everyone in the room knew what was going to happen. He was going to take a pain killer that would interact with the warfarin and suffer a catastrophic bleed.

So how did it happen? The patient saw a locum GP on a morning when the computer crashed. The locum didn't know him or ask about his other medications before giving him a prescription for a non-steroidal anti-inflammatory drug (NSAID). His usual pharmacy had a big Christmas queue so he went to an unfamiliar chemist who also didn't check his medications. And his blood test at the warfarin clinic was delayed because of the holidays. He went home, ate some turkey and had a massive stomach bleed.

Most examples showed how heavily GPs rely on their computer to prevent cock-ups, and how simply errors can occur. E.g., a consultant mumbled the name of a drug – triamcinolone – into a tape recorder and it was wrongly transcribed as methotrexate. Not even close. The letter was sent to the GP unchecked. The GP issued a prescription. The pharmacist queried it but was satisfied when the receptionist read the letter back to her. The drug was given as an injection by the practice nurse who didn't realise it was cytotoxic (i.e. able to kill healthy tissue) and got her decimal point in the wrong place, giving ten times the dose. The nurse realised her latter mistake, got the patient into A&E and reported the error. The Primary Care Trust has now banned cytotoxic injections in primary care and offered medicine safety training, which GPs are too busy to attend.

For patients, the best chance of avoiding drug errors is to know what drugs you're taking, what the side effects are and what you can, and can't, take with them. And check the name and dose with whoever is about to inject you. Avoiding misdiagnosis or substandard treatment is harder, but patients now have free access to the Map of Medicine via the NHS Choices website (www.nhs.uk). This is a superb distillation of the treatment you should be getting. If you ask nicely, your GP should be able to access it during the consultation, so you can prevent an error happening rather than join the 10% of patients who are harmed by their treatment[1].

To be continued . . .

---

[1] An estimate extrapolated from a few studies. No-one knows the true scale of medical error.

AFTERTHOUGHTS

AFTERTHOUGHTS

Has it been worth raking over the ashes of scandals past? So much good stuff goes on in the NHS, it doesn't seem terribly wise filling a whole book with the dark side of healthcare – a bit like a fruit salad made only of tomatoes. If we'd learned the lessons of Bristol and beyond, I'd happily shut up. But I still think we've a way to go before safety is given the priority it deserves in the NHS, and we owe it to those who've suffered in the masking (and unmasking) of these scandals not to keep repeating the same mistakes. Lord Darzi, who surely knows as much as anyone about the state of the NHS, told me he 'wasn't surprised' with the key finding of the *Why Children Die* report that 69% of deaths are (still) avoidable or potentially avoidable.

At least we're measuring bad outcomes, rather than hiding them, but the NHS can't improve unless the time and resources are dedicated to training and inspiring the staff, allowing them to work in teams that focus on the patient in front of them rather than the politician three hundred miles away. The NHS has certainly got much better since I qualified in 1987. The bastard surgeon has died out with the two-year waiting list, the quality of care has improved, treatments are more effective and there is far more scrutiny, teamwork and openness than there used to be.

However, it's sill a splintered and fractious organisation. Eighteen years after I tried it, junior doctors are still ripping into the Government and medical establishment for screwing up their training. RemedyUK, the voice of grass-roots doctors, is considering reporting the chief medical officer and other senior medical architects of Modernising Medical Careers to the GMC for enforcing an 'unsafe, defective and disastrous' scheme, despite clear warnings that it wouldn't work.

Many frontline staff remain vehemently opposed to the forced introduction of private competition into the NHS. Managers and clinical staff are at least united in their belief that politicians and the Department of Health still interfere far too much in the running of the NHS, but devolution can only occur if clinical staff take on more management responsibility and many prefer just to treat patients.

However well intentioned, centrally imposed reform of healthcare just doesn't work, particularly if the staff aren't involved in or inspired by it. What the NHS needs above all is a focus to unite around, something that everyone (politicians, managers, clinicians and support staff) can agree on.

Why not patient safety? Healthcare is unpredictable and we can never 'do no harm' to patients, but we could at least try to minimise it. And safe environments tend to be calmer and much more pleasant to work (and be sick) in, with fewer thrown scalpels and hissy fits, and more time to devote to compassion without the niggling worry that what you're giving (or getting) is sub standard care. This is far from straight-forward. For a start, you have to measure things that might show you're making patients worse rather than better. And bad news is far easier to hide than own up to.

Ernest Codman, the Boston surgeon of a century ago, was so disgusted with his colleagues at Massachusetts General Hospital putting 'income before outcome' that he resigned to set up his own 'End-Result' Hospital: 'Every hospital should follow every patient it treats, long enough to determine whether or not the treatment has been successful, and then to enquire "if not, why not?" with a view to preventing similar failures in the future.' Codman also believed in publishing and classifying adverse treatment, according to:

Lack of technical knowledge or skill
Lack of surgical judgement
Lack of care or equipment
Lack of diagnostic skill.

He also acknowledged that some patients didn't get better because they had unconquerable disease or simply refused treatment. And sometimes shit happened for reasons beyond anyone's control.

Codman was commendably open about his own errors – he once killed a patient by tying off his hepatic duct: 'an error of skill of the most gross character that even during the operation, I failed to recognise it'. But the fact that he was a surgeon brave enough to own up to his cockups earned him the right to kick medical ass. Without the scientific evaluation of outcomes, he concluded, there was nothing to distinguish a surgeon from 'a genial charlatan'.

Codman was initially ostracised and ridiculed by the medical establishment. However, he devised minimal standards for hospitals which were partially adopted by the American Surgical Society and are still relevant today. We have to measure and analyse outcomes to define minimal standards and we have to analyse individual errors and near misses to prevent them happening again. This applies as much to general practice as hospital care.

Safety should be central to the NHS but the fact that it isn't is partly due to its cost and difficulty. You start with a cash-strapped, under staffed, fire-fighting service full of high emotion, political interference and vested interests, where shit gets buried until the stench is too great to bear. Then you try to switch to a calm, well-resourced service where everyone admits to errors and works in teams, involving patients and giving and accepting scrutiny and feedback to anticipate and prevent harm. It takes money, leadership and training. The staff need to think about the service they're providing and how to make it better for patients, but the NHS has never set aside time to do this. We're always at the front line, always at war and flying by the seat of our pants.

A safety culture in the NHS requires a minimum of bureaucratic interference. This isn't to say that politicians don't have a role – they should be involved in setting standards and ensuring that the staff have the resources to meet them. Measuring outcomes is important, but you also need to think of the process too. One reason we need to centralise complex treatment in fewer sites is that we just don't have sufficient expertise or resources to support smaller units. Just by looking at outcomes, a small unit may appear to be coping, but when you turn over the stone and discover they've only got one consultant surgeon on-call around the clock, day in, day out, you know there's a disaster waiting to happen.

Similarly, some safety issues are common sense. You don't need to measure outcomes or perform a large trial to realise that all drugs shouldn't be stored in identical vials so they're easy to mix up in the heat of a cardiac arrest. Or that dangerous drugs should be left around on wards in which they're never needed. Or that obsolete anaesthetic machines deemed too dangerous for theatre shouldn't be used in casualty departments. It's taken the NHS a while to cotton onto this, but we're slowly getting more safety-conscious and more open about the dangers of medicine.

The key to openness is a swift explanation and apology to patients and relatives when things go wrong, plus appropriate compensation whatever the cause. Litigation would then become far less likely, except in cases of obvious negligence. More often disasters happen because of a chain of contributory factors, not the single action of one person (although all the doctors I know can think of errors for which they blame themselves). But the commonest response from patients and relatives after medical error is not to blame individuals, but for those involved and the wider NHS to learn from mistakes to stop them happening to someone else.

Lord Darzi recently invited me to his surgical unit at St Mary's and Imperial College in London, where he's been pioneering safety interventions based on what works in the airline industry. Initially he struggled against the defensive culture of the NHS. When black boxes were introduced into planes in the fifties, they caused outrage amongst pilots, many of whom threatened to go on strike. Fast-forward 40 years and Darzi, then a new surgical consultant, decided to introduce a black box in his operating theatre. This recorded the patient's vital signs, the anaesthetic procedures and, most contentiously, the surgical team, on video, as it went about its business.

Within 24 hours, someone had put bin liners over his cameras. But today, the black box is still up and running. His colleagues accept that the recorded information allows them to learn from near misses so that tragedies are avoided. Every surgeon gets into difficult situations, but the safe ones know how to get out of them.

Darzi enlisted a psychologist, Charles Vincent, to investigate the role of human factors in medical error. One of Vincent's approaches is to allow doctors to take time out to observe their colleagues going about their work and to suggest improvements. One junior doctor was so horrified about how unsafe handover was at the end of a shift that she devised a checklist to improve it.

Darzi has also developed a simulated operating theatre that teaches his team to manage common distractions (e.g. constant interruptions during surgery) and rare, life-threatening emergencies. Pilots are legally obliged to spend sixteen hours a year in a simulator, proving their competence to manage the worst-case scenarios, but for surgeons and anaesthetists, it is still optional.

Darzi is also helping to pioneer a surgical checklist with the World Health Organisation to ensure patients are given the appropriate drugs before surgery, that the right bit is being removed and that everyone is prepared for what might go wrong. This also encourages staff to speak up to protect patients. So how would Darzi react if a junior nurse told him he was about to operate on the wrong side? 'That would be the most refreshing thing ever.'

In his recent NHS review, Darzi announced that hospitals should no longer claim a fee for 'wrong site' surgery. Why were they ever allowed to? There are nearly 14,000 different diagnoses for which we now have successful treatments and they aren't going to go right all the time. But we shouldn't reward things that should never happen.

And we should keep encouraging staff to find their own solutions. In one American hospital with a seemingly intractable MRSA problem, a new manager decided to stop shouting at the staff and start listening to them. They devised their own plan (e.g. a stethoscope for each patient, keeping the common equipment you might need by each bed) and cut the infection rate by 85%.

For the NHS to embrace safety, politicians must recognise that it's not how quickly you get treated that matters, but how safely. Rushing to hit targets can make you cut corners. Depending on whose figures you believe, between 25,000 and 40,000 patients die each year in the NHS from avoidable errors, the equivalent of a jumbo jet crashing each week. But not everyone accepts change. Some doctors think checklists reduce them to factory workers, others have a tantrum if someone reminds them to wash their hands. If you're looking for a safe hospital, it's more likely to be one that reports more errors. The hospital that admits to nothing generally has the most to hide.

The NHS has made some progress in identifying and learning from individual errors, particularly where it's obvious that the wrong thing has been done (wrong diagnosis, wrong drug, wrong kidney). But until we rationalise complex surgery to fewer units and enforce a statistical standard that identifies and investigates dangerous units, we can't say NHS surgery is safe. Let's hope the Care Quality Commission has the independence and influence to do this.

We also need minimal standards for process, to ensure all units have the staff, resources and facilities to provide treatment safely. After the Bristol heart scandal, the Paediatric Cardiac Services Review concluded that child heart surgery should be centralised to fewer (e.g. six) centres to concentrate expertise and resources. There were (and are) shortages of specialist nurses, anaesthetists, cardiologists, surgeons and perfusionists, so it would be safer for patients to travel further to a larger, well-staffed unit. However, the Government rejected this because there were no statistically poor units and they didn't want the political flak of having to close down units.

When I met Bruce Keogh at the NICE conference in December 2007, he told me that there were still thirteen paediatric cardiac centres and three were down to a single consultant surgeon. How can that be safe? Perfusionists, who have the complex and vital job of operating the heart bypass machines, are also in short supply and are expected to miraculously cover both adults and children requiring bypass surgery. In May 2005, five-month-old Abbie Hattam died following an accidental drug overdose given by a very stressed, over worked perfusionist during open heart surgery in Bristol. The coroner's verdict was one of unlawful killing. A subsequent investigation identified both the regulation and shortage of perfusionists as key factors in Abbie's death. The fact they still aren't regulated a decade after the disastrous death of Hannah Shepherd at Guy's Hospital in 1998 is beyond belief.

Labour's failure to centralise child heart surgery has compounded the shortage of perfusionists. This unacceptable risk to patients prompted the resignation of Bristol surgeon Ash Pawade, who did more than anyone to turn around the unit in its darkest hour and achieved exceptionally good results under great pressure. Pawade claims the United Bristol Healthcare Trust tried to prevent him from publicising the staff shortages that made his working environment intolerable. The Trust denies the claims but it doesn't sound like the mature, calm atmosphere where safety can flourish.

So I've ended up back where I started, exposing scandals in Bristol. At least we investigate now after one unexpected death, rather than 35. But while specialist surgery is stretched across too many centres and no-one is brave enough to define safe processes and outcomes, we can't just blithely say that 'all surgery is safe'. Safety, and its big brother quality, have the potential to unite the NHS, but they're still being buried under bureaucratic guff and political cowardice. Maybe it would help if patients waved their arms about a bit.

THE CONSCIOUS PATIENT GUIDE

Why is it taking the NHS so long to get better? One reason is that, for much of its 60 years, it just hasn't had the resources to provide a fully comprehensive, high-quality service free-at-the-front-door. According to the Wanless Report, between 1972 and 1998 underinvestment in the NHS compared to the EU average came to £276 billion. So it's going to take a decade of sustained and sensible investment to get it back on track.

But it needs more than money. It needs politicians at the top to unite around safety and patients sitting the bottom to find their voice. The bottom line of this book is that the NHS has a long way to go before we can take safety as a given. But you can help by asking questions. You may not get the answer you want, or you may not get any answer at all, but for the culture of the NHS to become more open, we have to mean it when we ask: 'Have you got any questions?'

A lot of people feel much happier trusting NHS staff to get on with their jobs without having to check up on them, and that's fine. When you're sick, you often don't have the energy to object. Just remember – there is no such thing as a stupid question. And if you don't understand the answer, keep asking it until you do.

How to Get the Right Treatment

This is surprisingly difficult. It helps if you have the right diagnosis and that often depends on being given the time to tell your story. Also, you may find that the best treatment according to the evidence just makes you feel dreadful. If you do get unpleasant side-effects, you can report them at www.yellowcard.gov.uk. This scheme is vital to monitoring the safety of all drugs, particularly new ones. You can also report dangerous incidents to National Patient Safety Agency (www.npsa.nhs.uk/nrls/reporting/) – although they won't investigate individual concerns – and you can get authoritative information about any drug at www.bnf.org.uk – although you may have to pretend you work in the NHS to register.

People are genetically different and respond differently to drugs, no matter what the trial evidence predicts. Patients also have different priorities depending on what they value most. As a junior doctor, I met a woman with cervical cancer whose surgeon was very keen for her to have a hysterectomy to reduce the risk of it coming back. But she was keen to have a more local operation to give her the best chance of having children, even if the risk of recurrence was greater. Such complex decisions can only be made if patients are encouraged to participate.

A lot also depends on how information is presented to you. Say you've had a heart attack or suffer from angina and you want to reduce your risk of dying from heart disease. A doctor might say: 'I think a cholesterol-lowering drug is a good thing,' and leave it at that. But if you asked how likely the treatment was to help you, in numerical terms, there are lots of ways the information could be phrased:

'If you take this drug every day for five years, your risk of death will be reduced by nearly 40%.'

'If you take this drug every day for five years, your risk of death will fall from 8% to 5%.'

'If 33 people like you take this drug every day for five years, one death will be prevented but I don't know whether it will be yours.'

'If you swallowed 1,825 tablets of this drug at a
rate of one a day for five years and at a
prescription cost of £426, your risk of death
would fall by 0.9%. The recognised side-effects are
muscle damage, headache, abdominal pain,
nausea, vomiting, hairloss, anaemia, dizziness,
depression, nerve damage, hepatitis, jaundice,
pancreatitis and hypersensitivity syndrome.'

Which of the statements is most likely to convince you to take
the drug? In fact, all the statements are about the same statin
but the first – the relative risk reduction – is the one most
quoted in press releases, advertisements and newspaper
headlines. Naturally, the drug companies are keen to hype up
the benefits and doctors may put a positive slant on prescribing
some drugs because we get paid to hit targets. Asking for the
absolute, as well as the relative, risk-reduction is a good way of
getting the benefits of a treatment in perspective.

Another way of understanding how effective a treatment
might be is to ask about the Number Needed to Treat (NNT)
to prevent one whatever it is you're trying to avoid (death, a
heart attack, a stroke). This again can be a bit dispiriting
because often, particularly in prevention, we have to treat a
hundred or more patients for a year to prevent one nasty thing
happening to one of them. When you tell patients the odds,
many decide that their risk is small and they'd rather not take
the tablets.

Similarly, the Number Needed to Harm is the number of
patients who can have a treatment before one gets a nasty side-
effect, and the Number Needed to Screen is the number of
people who have to have screening to save one life or stop one
nasty event (e.g. case of cervical cancer). For screening, the
numbers are often very large and you may end up thinking
'why bother?' but no-one can foresee what will happen to you

as an individual and how much medical intervention you opt for depends largely on your attitude to risk.

And to show you're really on the ball, you could ask how reliable the evidence is to support the information you've been given. Most research still concentrates on death and disease, rather than how you feel after treatment, and the strength of evidence falls broadly into four categories, from good (A) to poor (D).

A. Evidence derived from randomised controlled trials (RCTs) or systematic reviews of RCTs (e.g. a meta-analysis)
B. Evidence from non-randomised trials or observational studies
C. Professional consensus
D. Individual opinion.

In much of surgery, the standard of proof is still poor and you have to make decisions based on personal opinion – so remember, the more doctors you see, the more opinions you'll get. For medical treatments, there should be better trial evidence on which to base your judgement.

If you like short cuts, you could ask what treatment your doctor would recommend for his mother or daughter. Some doctors prefer not to make any recommendations, but give you the figures and leave the choice up to you. If you want to know what it means to have a particular illness and what treatment has in store for you, there's an excellent website, www.healthtalkonline.org, with videos and transcripts of interviews with patients and carers, and help with how to make sense of the complex choices offered to you.

The Ottawa Personal Decision Guide is another good place to start. It prompts you to consider precisely what the decision you need to make is, how certain you are about the benefits and risks of each option, what additional information you need and what outcome matters most to you. You can download the generic guide and a selection of aids for specific decisions, at http://decisionaid.ohri.ca/index.html

When a patient asks me a question and I'm stuck for the answer, I usually log onto www.gpnotebook.co.uk, which you can access free. The *British Medical Journal* has a best treatments website (http://besttreatments.bmj.com/) which you have to subscribe to (but you can get it free via the Boots website if you don't mind the adverts – www.askboots health.com). NHS Choices (www.nhs.uk) has lots of free information, including the fabulous Map of Medicine. And NICE publishes summaries just for patients that they're desperate for you to read and then demand the treatment you deserve (www.nice.org.uk). The new NHS Constitution gives every patient who needs it the right to receive NICE-approved treatment (and NICE approves far more drugs than it doesn't). It'll be interesting to see how this works in practice.

If you'd like to record your experiences of the NHS on-line, and check out other people's, there are two websites – www.patientopinion.org.uk (which concentrates on the overall treatment) and www.Iwantgreatcare.org (which invites you to rate individual doctors). The trick with feedback is to try to write something positive first, if you can, and then offer constructive suggestions for improvement.

Some doctors aren't terribly keen on these sites, worried that they might be used by vexatious patients to settle scores when doctors are unable to respond because they're bound by confidentiality. Professor Chris Bulstrode, a high-profile supporter, predicted 'a few doctors might be caught with their trousers down.' A review (now deleted) of a consultant psychiatrist seemed to bear this out: 'He put his wanger in my ear. I'm not a psychiatric case. He did it twice. NO COMPUNCTION AT ALL.'

Experience of similar sites in America suggests most patients take a useful and constructive approach. But it's even better to try to interact during your consultations, to prevent problems happening in the first place. It's tough if you've done a lot of background reading only to be met with a surly, uncooperative doctor or nurse. The NHS needs to be open not just about its results, but in its attitude.

It's even tougher if you've spent a lot of time researching a particular drug or treatment and then find out your local NHS won't fund it. There are lots of issues here, ranging from the prohibitive cost of new drugs (when shareholders are involved, profitability is the prime motivating force, which is why a market system will never provide cheaper healthcare) to the lengthy appraisal process NICE uses and then the wilful disregard of NICE guidance once it has been issued. There are still gross postcode lotteries in the UK – not only do the four countries have different drug policies but there are huge variations in whether those policies are implemented.

In England some PCTs stick strictly to NICE guidance, others allow drugs to be used before NICE has made a decision, and some doctors completely disregard the guidance of both NICE and their PCT to use their own judgement to decide what's best for patients. The result is that two people with the same condition living in the same street can still get very different treatment. Patients can appeal if a drug is denied, but most appeals are turned down.

Maybe the NHS should make its own drugs. At the very least, the Government should put pressure on drug companies to reduce their prices and allow patients to top up their treatment with drugs that it can't or won't fund. Rationing, and the fact that some people have more money than others, are both facts of life and promoting patient choice while denying the dying a shot at a new cancer or Alzheimer's drug is absurd.

GETTING THE RIGHT
TREATMENT DONE RIGHT

This is tricky because it requires you to enquire about the competence of who's treating you, which doesn't always make for a cosy doctor – patient relationship. However, units with nothing to hide should be very open and forthcoming about their methods and their results. If you can get the hang of asking for specialist centres where large numbers of patients are treated, information about standards, access to audit that shows these standards have been met and a guarantee that trainee staff will be adequately supervised, you'll have done a lot to ensure you get a good standard of care. And you'll keep shifting the culture from simplistic, paternalistic reassurance to a meeting between experts.

If you're having surgery, you can download the WHO surgical safety checklist at www.who.int/patientsafety/safe surgery/tools_resources/SSSL_Checklist_finalJun08.pdf

Before you have your anaesthetic, the surgical team should all agree on your identity, the site of the surgery, the procedure to be performed and whether you've given your consent, but it might be possible for you to join in this pre-briefing session and meet the team. You could check that the right side has been marked up and that everyone knows about your allergies. You could also check that you're going to get antibiotics to prevent infections and drugs to prevent you getting a deep vein thrombosis. Thousands of people die unnecessarily each year because they weren't given treatment to prevent DVTs, which are common after surgery and bed rest, and can break off and cause pulmonary embolism. So it can't harm to enquire about prophylaxis.

Think of yourself as an inquisitive child. Ask about all the gadgets and bits of tubing. You probably should have a pulse oximeter put on a finger to measure the percentage of your haemoglobin that is saturated with oxygen. Have you? And is it working? What's the reading now? Remember, there's no such thing as a stupid question.

It isn't easy asking challenging questions when you're ill and anxious. Perhaps the best surgery short cut is to track down a theatre nurse and ask which surgeon she would choose (or rather whom she would avoid). Another option is to compile a list of questions you might like to ask in advance, and then pick a few that take your fancy. Here's a list of questions you could ask any doctor:

- What do you think is wrong with me?
- What tests will I need?
- What do the tests involve?
- When will I know the results?
- What treatments are there to choose from?
- What are the risks and benefits of the different options?
- Will the treatment effect my work, study, sex or social life?
- How long will the treatment last?
- How do I know if I'm getting the best treatment?
- Will I be able to look after my family or will I need help?
- Will the treatment affect my fertility?
- Will I be able to drive?
- How can I tell my family and friends?
- Would you like a chocolate?

Here are some slightly more 'on the nose' questions which suggest you've done a bit of homework:

- Are you a specialist?

- How many of this particular type of operation have you done?
- If a junior surgeon is doing my operation, will he be closely supervised by a specialist?
- What have your results been in the long term?
- What standard are you auditing your work against?
- Do you have any published audits you could show me?
- How does it compare to the national average?
- How likely is it that this treatment will improve the length or quality of my life?
- How likely is it that this treatment will harm me? How?
- Can you give me numerical risks, rather than just platitudes?
- How confident are you of those figures?
- Is there another unit in the NHS that gets much better results than yours?
- Would you like a chocolate? Not the purple one, that's my favourite.

Some hospitals already publish excellent patient information packs that suggest and invite questions, but not all. Some also show patients an analysis of their results routinely, without you having to feel awkward by asking for them. To give informed consent, you need information and perhaps the biggest sign that the culture of medicine has changed would be if the information was always given upfront with a smile instead of you having to drag it out of a surly nurse.

Finally, it's worth doing a few safety checks as you go along. So feel free to ask:

- Is that bag of blood really for me? Do you mind if we check?
- How fast should the bag run through? It was eight-hourly yesterday.

- What are these large purple tablets? I normally have small white ones.
- Would you like a grape? Would you mind washing your hands first?

We can probably learn from America here too. Ernest Codman's minimal standards for surgery ran until 1952, when they were consumed by an organisation now known as the Joint Commission on Accreditation of Healthcare Organizations (JCACHO).

JCACHO is similar to our Care Quality Commission but with bigger and better-established balls. It's an independent, not-for-profit organisation, that accredits and certifies more than 15,000 healthcare organisations in the United States. It's mission is to continuously improve the safety and quality of care (if you're lucky enough to have insurance).

Now here's the interesting part. The commission sees active and involved patients as vital to driving up standards in healthcare. Research has shown that patients who take part in decisions about their healthcare are more likely to get better faster. And one way to reduce errors and improve outcomes is to ask questions. The commission has even printed out the kind of questions you might like to ask as part of its Speak Up campaign. On pages 314–18 are examples of questions for hospital care.

Getting patients to closely monitor their own treatment and safety may lead to a bit of conflict on the wards and in the surgery, and as an approach it's still being evaluated. But the reported error rates in US hospitals do seem to be lower than in the UK and it may be because the staff take safety more seriously (possibly because they're petrified of being sued). Lord Darzi has spotted this intervention too and runs video clips on his wards encouraging patients to speak up if they spot anything untoward (e.g. a professor of surgery forgetting to wash his hands).

You may feel a bit shy about doing this, so first cut out and fill in your Royal College of Patients membership card (see page 321) and have it on display. Then ask a question. Go on, be brave. You are a vice president, after all. And, if you're feeling particularly keen, you could write about your experience on patientopinion.org.uk or Iwantgreatcare.org. Your story might even change the NHS, or at least make it easier for someone else. But remember, positive points first. The staff need all the encouragement they can get. If you really can't think of anything constructive to write, please send it to *Private Eye*.

SPEAK UP QUESTIONS
ADAPTED SLIGHTLY FROM THE JOINT COMMISSION
www.jointcommission.org

Speak up if you have questions or concerns. If you still don't understand, ask again. It's your body and you have a right to know.

- Your health is very important. Do not worry about being embarrassed if you don't understand something that your doctor, nurse or other healthcare professional tells you. If you don't understand because you speak another language, ask for someone who speaks your language. You have the right to get free help from someone who speaks your language.
- Don't be afraid to ask about safety. If you're having surgery, ask the doctor to mark the area that is to be operated on.
- Don't be afraid to tell the nurse or the doctor if you think you are about to get the wrong medicine.
- Don't be afraid to tell a healthcare professional if you think he or she has confused you with another patient.

Pay attention to the care you get. Always make sure you're getting the right treatments and medicines by the right healthcare professionals. Don't assume anything.

- Tell your nurse or doctor if something doesn't seem right.
- Expect healthcare workers to introduce themselves. Look for their identification (ID) badges. A new mother should know the person she hands her baby to. If you don't know who the person is, ask for their ID.
- Notice whether your caregivers have washed their hands.

Hand washing is the most important way to prevent infections. Don't be afraid to remind a doctor or nurse to do this.

- Know what time of the day you normally get medicine. If you don't get it, tell your nurse or doctor.
- Make sure your nurse or doctor checks your ID. Make sure he or she checks your wristband and asks your name before he or she gives you your medicine or treatment.

Educate yourself about your illness. Learn about the medical tests you get, and your treatment plan.

- Ask your doctor about the special training and experience that qualifies him or her to treat your illness.
- Look for information about your condition. Good places to get that information are from your doctor, your library, respected websites and support groups.
- Write down important facts your doctor tells you. Ask your doctor if he or she has any written information you can keep.
- Read all medical forms and make sure you understand them before you sign anything. If you don't understand, ask your doctor or nurse to explain them.
- Make sure you know how to work any equipment that is being used in your care. If you use oxygen at home, do not smoke or let anyone smoke near you.

Ask a trusted family member or friend to be your advocate (adviser or supporter).

- Your advocate can ask questions that you may not think about when you are stressed.
- Ask this person to stay with you, even overnight, when you are hospitalised. You will be able to rest better. Your advocate can help make sure you get the right medicines and treatments.

- Your advocate can also help remember answers to questions you have asked. He or she can speak up for you when you cannot speak up for yourself.
- Make sure this person understands the kind of care you want. Make sure he or she knows what you want done about life support and other life-saving efforts if you are unconscious and not likely to get better.
- Go over the consents for treatment with your advocate before you sign them. Make sure you both understand exactly what you are about to agree to.
- Make sure your advocate understands the type of care you will need when you get home. Your advocate should know what to look for if your condition is getting worse. He or she should also know whom to call for help.

Know what medicines you take and why you take them. Medicine errors are the most common healthcare mistakes.

- Ask about why you should take the medication. Ask for written information about it, including its brand and generic names. Also ask about the side-effects of all medicines.
- If you do not recognise a medicine, double-check that it is for you. Ask about medicines that you are to take by mouth before you swallow them. Read the contents of the bags of intravenous (IV) fluids. If you're not well enough to do this, ask your advocate to do it.
- If you are given an IV, ask the nurse how long it should take for the liquid to run out. Tell the nurse if it doesn't seem to be dripping right (too fast or too slow).
- Whenever you get a new medicine, tell your doctors and nurses about allergies you have, or negative reactions you have had to other medicines.
- If you are taking a lot of medicines, be sure to ask your doctor or pharmacist if it is safe to take those medicines

together. Do the same thing with vitamins, herbs and over-the-counter drugs.

- Make sure you can read the handwriting on prescriptions written by your doctor. If you can't read it, the pharmacist may not be able to either. Ask somebody at the doctor's office to print the prescription, if necessary.
- Carry an up-to-date list of the medicines you are taking in your purse or wallet. Write down how much you take and when you take it. Go over the list with your doctor and other caregivers.

Use a hospital, clinic, surgery centre, or other type of healthcare organisation that has been carefully checked out. For example, the Healthcare Commission (now part of the Care Quality Commission) visits hospitals to see if they are meeting quality standards. Ask to see the latest inspection report.

- Ask about the healthcare organisation's experience in taking care of people with your type of illness. How often do they perform the procedure you need? What special care do they provide to help patients get well?
- If you have more than one hospital to choose from, ask your doctor which one has the best care for your condition.
- Before you leave the hospital or other facility, ask about follow-up care and make sure that you understand all of the instructions.
- Go to the Healthcare Commission at www.healthcarecommission.org.uk and read more about the patient safety and quality standards at all the hospitals or clinics you could choose from.

Participate in all decisions about your treatment. You are the centre of the healthcare team.

- You and your doctor should agree on exactly what will be done during each step of your care.
- Know who will be taking care of you. Know how long the treatment will last. Know how you should feel.
- Understand that more tests or medications may not always be better for you. Ask your doctor how a new test or medication will help.
- Keep copies of your medical records from previous hospital stays and share them with your healthcare team. This will give them better information about your health history.
- Don't be afraid to ask for a second opinion. If you are unsure about the best treatment for your illness, talk with one or two additional doctors. The more information you have about all the kinds of treatment available to you, the better you will feel about the decisions made.
- Ask to speak with others who have had the same treatment or operation you may have to have. They may help you prepare for the days and weeks ahead. They may be able to tell you what to expect and what worked best for them.
- Talk to your doctor and your family about your wishes regarding resuscitation and other life-saving actions.

HARSH TRUTHS

There are lots of harsh truths about healthcare. Doctors are human. We make mistakes. Half of us are below average. Some nurses are ruder than others. People are living longer. The rich live even longer. There's still plenty we can't cure. Death is part of living. Shit happens. Some drugs are ridiculously expensive. They don't work as well as the manufacturers claim. The NHS can't afford every treatment. The NHS wastes a lot of our money. Patients don't take their tablets. Patients are human too.

You can ignore harsh truths and hope they don't all creep up on you at the same time. Or you can try to minimise their impact. No-one has come up with a fair way of slicing up the NHS cake, and all health services have to ration healthcare. We'd need to ration it less if we didn't squander so much money on endless reorganisation, energy wastage, ineffective treatment, substandard care and avoidable error. Like a very large tablet, this book isn't easy to swallow in one go, and if the outcome is just to provide fodder for politicians to push through their reforms and try to control the NHS from the centre, then I will have made the health service worse, rather than better. But if I've encouraged just a few patients to ask questions, I may have done some good.

Whether you want to ask questions or not, you're now expected to answer them. 'What distance would you be prepared to travel for surgery at a hospital with half the mortality rate of your local hospital?' and 'How much would you be willing to pay for an extra year of good-quality life?' These questions aren't coming soon, they're out there already. It's our health service, and it'll only get better if we get involved.

FURTHER READING

Patient Safety by Charles Vincent (Churchill Livingstone) is a wise, balanced, insightful and motivating overview. I should have read it earlier.

Better and *Complications*, two books by American surgeon Atul Gawande (Profile), are gripping and humane accounts of the complexity, triumphs and challenges of healthcare. Gawande opts for understanding rather than exposure, and promotes positive deviancy rather than nihilistic ranting. I fear he may have a point.

How Shall I Tell the Dog? by Miles Kington (also Profile) is an object lesson in how to die with style and humour, and how to make death earn its living.

CUT OUT AND KEEP

THE ROYAL COLLEGE OF PATIENTS
Vice President

DR PHIL

Phil Hammond is a GP, writer, comic and broadcaster. He has worked in sexual health and as a lecturer in medical communication at two universities (Birmingham and Bristol). He currently works part-time as a GP and will continue until the GMC tells him to stop. Phil is still *Private Eye*'s medical correspondent and possibly the only comedian to have appeared at a Public Inquiry. He has been a regular panellist on *Have I Got News for You*, *The News Quiz*, *The Now Show* and *Countdown*, and presented five series of *Trust Me, I'm a Doctor* on BBC2. Dr Phil is a Patron of the Herpes Viruses Association and a Vice President of both the Patients' Association and the Royal College of Patients. He has written one other book, *Medicine Balls*, which is much funnier but still vaguely serious.